My Life in Pursuit of
Exceptional Physical Fitness

My Life in Pursuit of Exceptional Physical Fitness

AGES SIX TO SEVENTY-THREE...AND COUNTING

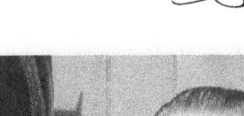

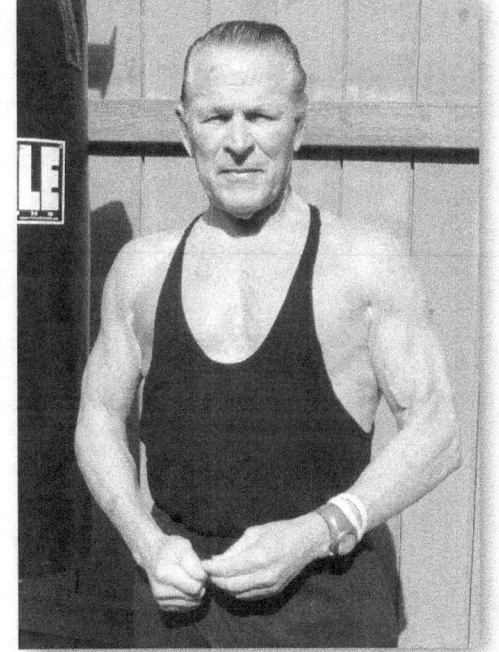

Phillip Dan Cook, PhD, ACE, NASM

ISBN: 1543001297
ISBN 13: 9781543001297
Library of Congress Control Number: 2017902047
CreateSpace Independent Publishing Platform
North Charleston, South Carolina

Disclaimer

THIS BOOK IS INTENDED SOLELY for information and educational purposes and does not constitute medical advice. Please consult a medical or health professional before you begin any exercise, nutrition, or supplementation program or if you have questions about your health.

For people in poor health or with preexisting physical or mental health conditions, there may be risks associated with participating in activities or using products mentioned in this book. Because these risks exist, you should not use the products or participate in the activities described in this book if you are in poor health or if you have a preexisting mental or physical health condition. If you choose to participate in these activities, you do so knowingly and voluntarily of your own free will and accord, assuming all risks associated with these activities.

While all attempts have been made to verify the information provided in this publication, neither the author nor the publisher assumes any responsibility for errors, omissions, or contrary interpretations of the subject matter herein. This book is for entertainment purposes only. The views expressed are those of the author alone and should not be taken as expert instruction or commands. The reader is responsible for his or her own actions. Adherence to all applicable laws and regulations—including international, federal, state, and local laws governing professional licensing, business practices, advertising, and all other aspects of doing business in the United States, Canada, the United Kingdom, or any other jurisdiction—is the sole responsibility of the purchaser or reader. Neither the author nor the publisher assumes any responsibility or liability whatsoever on the behalf of the purchaser or reader of these materials. Any perceived slight of any individual or organization is purely unintentional.

I would like to dedicate this book to two of our pugs, *Harley-Man and Honey Pearl*, who spent many hours comforting me as I struggled to write this book. Certainly, Harley-Man will be a major character in my next book, *Our Dogs.* Honey Pearl will also be in the book but unfortunately she had a seizer while being treated for pancreatitis and passed away. *So, so sad for a very sweet, young pug!*

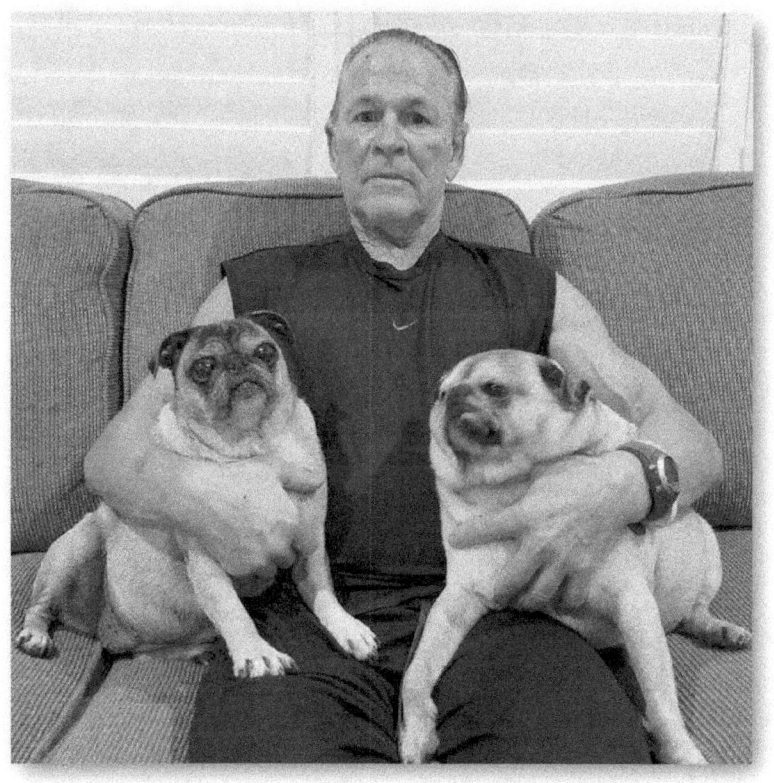

Contents

PART 1

Introduction

CHAPTER 1 - WHY THIS BOOK? WHOM IS THIS BOOK FOR? WHAT THIS BOOK IS NOT!

THERE ARE FEW ACTIVITIES THAT we can track throughout our lives. Doing so is particularly difficult with activities that change as we age. Our personal level of physical fitness is an activity that can be measured. However, few people track their physical fitness throughout their lives. This book provides a detailed account of my *personal pursuit of exceptional physical fitness for sixty-seven years (from ages six to seventy-three) and counting)*.

I describe interesting, humorous, real-life physical fitness endeavors that I pursued in my early days and move on to my current physical activities to provide inspirational encouragement for young and older people to pursue a healthy life.

This is certainly not a book by a physical fitness scientist at the doctoral level trying to transfer highly technical information to the common person who wants to be physically fit. A number of books already provide highly technical information about specific and general aspects of physical fitness. There are books on heart rates, cardio training, strength training, and literally hundreds more topics.

This book covers the *essential aspects* that one would pursue to obtain *exceptional physical fitness.*

A distinguishing aspect of my *pursuit of exceptional physical fitness* is that I have continued to increase my physical activities as I age. Typically, one's physical fitness efforts decrease as he or she ages.

I describe what I now do based on research, observations of others during their training, and years of experimenting with exceptional physical fitness endeavors. I also describe some elastic material movements I do that are novel, or certainly not practiced at my health club.

Overall, this is an account of how I did it: I did it my way.

One of my heroes is fitness expert *Jack LaLanne*. When asked how old he wanted to be, LaLanne responded, *"I don't care how old I live! I just want to be living while I am living!"*

I believe it's never too late to do just that.

CHAPTER 2 - WHO AM I?

I AM A PHYSICAL FITNESS nut and have been my whole life. Maybe I inherited this from my father, or maybe this is just the way I turned out. I have combined my physical fitness endeavors with an intense, successful career in drug-discovery science. However, in this book, I focus on my physical fitness activities from age six to the present. I describe important aspects of my fitness endeavors and indicate which ones I believe were most effective in my *pursuit of exceptional physical fitness.* I also describe a fitness challenge in which I compare myself to *physical fitness "king" Jack LaLanne.*

I do not have a degree in exercise physiology or kinesiology. However, I do have a *PhD in medicinal chemistry*, and I have spent *fifty-two years of my life in drug discovery science.* I also have several prestigious physical fitness certifications, including certifications from the American Council on Exercise (***ACE***) and the National Academy of Sports Medicine (***NASM***). I have specialized in the older population and have trained older people at fitness clubs, clients' homes, and my own home.

In 2016, I stepped away from an exceptional scientific career. ***I have published over 250 scientific papers, and I am an inventor or coinventor of over 350 patents.***

Because of my exceptional career in drug-discovery science, another book may be in order. For sure, other scientists have met or exceeded my level of accomplishment. However, I am not aware of any high-level scientist who can compete with my ***sixty-seven years of pursuing exceptional physical fitness.***

The following passage is from a physical fitness brochure I was using several years ago:

I am a midseventies retired drug-discovery executive, senior research director, and entrepreneur in the areas of anticancer and anti-infective drugs (pancreatic and liver cancer, HIV, and HCV) with a doctorate in medicinal chemistry. I am also a lifelong fitness advocate. Although I have hypertension, arthritic knees, prostate problems, and exercise-induced asthma, I still aggressively pursue running and biking, resistance training, boxing workouts, and optimal nutrition and supplementation. I am a personal fitness trainer certified by the ***ACE*** (American Council on Exercise) and the ***NASM*** (National Academy of Sports Medicine). My continuing education has been focused on working with older adults, including frail, unhealthy adults, and this is the group of people I primarily focus on. I will train them individually or in small groups in their homes, my home, an appropriate club, or a medical facility. I will provide a free assessment of your fitness in the following areas:

- upper and lower body strength
- flexibility
- aerobic endurance
- motor ability
- dynamic balance
- posture analysis
- percent body fat

Your results will be compared with national ranges, which will indicate how you match up with your age group and provide a starting point to monitor subsequent fitness training that I will provide. I can guarantee that you will reach any goal you set for yourself!

To examine my own physical fitness level, I have taken the assessments noted above. In all areas, my scores were significantly better than those of individuals in their fifties. ***Chapter 5*** provides the results of other physical fitness tests I have taken.

Exceptional physical fitness embodies an effective diet, appropriate intake of vitamins and minerals, use of various supplements, cardio and strength training, stretching, and balance movements, all of which are discussed.

There are numerous ways to do cardio and strength training. Those described in this book are the ones that I have used, modified, invented, and found to be of value to my physical fitness.

PART 2

Physical Fitness

CHAPTER 3 - WHAT IS PHYSICAL FITNESS?

THERE ARE MANY DESCRIPTIONS OF physical fitness; they essentially note the same points. Several general descriptions are noted below.

Physical exercise is any bodily activity that enhances or maintains physical fitness and overall health and wellness. It is performed for various reasons, including strengthening the muscles and the cardiovascular system and honing athletic skills. Others engage in exercise for weight loss or maintenance or for mere enjoyment. Frequent and regular exercise boosts the immune system and helps prevent the so-called diseases of affluence: heart disease, cardiovascular disease, type 2 diabetes, and obesity. It may also help prevent stress and depression, promote or maintain positive self-esteem, and improve mental health generally. Childhood obesity is a growing global concern, and physical exercise may help decrease some of the effects of childhood and adult obesity. Some care providers call exercise a miracle drug or a wonder drug, alluding to the wide variety of benefits it can provide.

Fitness refers to the ability to perform physical activity. It also means having the energy and strength to feel as good as possible. Physical fitness is a general state of health and well-being and, more specifically, the ability to perform aspects of sports or occupations. Older adults will benefit from regular cardiovascular and strength training sessions, flexibility, and weight managing, just like anyone else. Indeed, older adults *need* exercise to forestall or even reverse some of the undesirable effects of being an older adult. Getting more fit, even a little bit, can improve your life. Research has suggested that just fifteen minutes each day can lengthen your life by three years. Exercise helps reduce blood pressure, maintain weight, stabilize blood sugar, and fight depression.

The list of the benefits of exercise continues to grow each year as researchers make more discoveries about how the human body works and the integral part exercise plays in overall health and wellness.

Physical fitness is generally achieved through a combination of cardio-respiratory efforts, strength training, wise nutrition, stretching, and balance movements. All these help you resist a sedentary lifestyle and the resulting hypokinetic diseases.

Hypokinetic diseases are conditions that occur from obesity and a sedentary lifestyle. *Hypo* means "less," and *kinetic* means "movement," so *hypokinetic* diseases are caused by a lack of physical activity. Hypokinetic conditions could include cardiovascular disease, some forms of cancer, back problems, obesity, type 2 diabetes, osteoporosis, mental health problems, high blood pressure, and heart disease.

A recent large study confirms that exercise lowers the risk of thirteen different types of cancer. According to the results of a pooled analysis of data from more than a million Europeans and Americans, higher levels of leisure-time physical activity are associated with a significantly lower risk of developing some types of cancer. For that group of thirteen cancers, the risk reduction ranged from 10 percent to 42 percent, and the overall average of the decrease of the select cancers was 16 percent.

Studies have suggested that people who are physically active "have lower rates of Alzheimer's and other age-associated neurodegenerative disorders."

As we age, the hippocampus—an area of our brains that is key to memory—shrinks, leading to memory problems and possibly dementia.

Research has shown that when previously sedentary men and women fifty to eighty years old walked around a track for forty minutes a day three times a week for six months, their hippocampi actually increased in size. A control group that did not walk had smaller hippocampi than when they started.

Another study of men and women with an average age of seventy-one found that those who had exercised moderately or vigorously over five years—jogging, hiking, swimming, or dancing—performed on a par with someone a decade younger on tests of memory and other brain skills. These studies support the prevailing theory that heart health and brain health are linked. Regular exercise helps prevent high blood pressure and stiffening of the arteries, and keeping blood vessels healthy ensures an optimal flow of blood to the brain. In addition, aerobic exercise creates higher levels of a protein known as brain-derived neurotrophic factor, or BDNF, which helps repair and protect the brain.

Strength training seems to help by sending pulses of blood into the brain. A study found that women who did moderate strength training at least once a week showed a 15 percent improvement on mental-skills tests.

So what does all this mean for those concerned about developing Alzheimer's? A recent study of men and women aged sixty-five or older found that those who were more active had a 50 percent reduced risk of developing the disease.

I certainly believe that cardio and strength training are essential aspects of physical fitness, ***but as I will describe later, my approach to exceptional physical fitness is to separate the two.***

CHAPTER 4 - WHAT IS EXCEPTIONAL PHYSICAL FITNESS?

I'M NOT SURE THERE IS a precise definition of exceptional physical fitness, but I am certain that it changes with age. In this chapter, I provide some comments on why I think I have not only pursued physical fitness but actually **been exceptionally physical fit throughout my life.**

I believe ***exceptional physical fitness*** is a combination of cardio and strength training. However, in this regard, I do not consider **Arnold Schwarzenegger** - one of my lifetime heroes - and other world-class body-builders to be exceptionally fit, as typically these athletes do little if any serious cardiorespiratory training. Likewise, on the other side, I do not consider **Lance Armstrong**—another of my heroes—to be in any way advanced in strength training. Similarly, I do not consider world-class marathoners to be physically fit overall, as these athletes do little strength training. Triathletes and decathletes may be considered better examples of physically fit people, as they require high levels of strength and cardiorespiratory fitness. Also, I do not believe the fitness craze of CrossFit is a good example for physical fitness. I will comment on this later.

In my early days, I was active and quite successful in sports (football, basketball, boxing, distance running, duathlons, and triathlons). In all these sports, *I was at the front of the line, for my father had pushed me to be the best.* Thus, I was the starting quarterback and safety and returned punts and kickoffs in football (junior high, high school, and junior college) and was a starting point guard in basketball (junior high and high school). I also anchored the mile medley relay team (ran the last half mile) in high school. We beat the state record several times during the season.

In junior college, I fought in the lightweight class *in the open division in the yearly New Mexico Golden Gloves Tournament.* I pushed hard to get my weight up to 165 for my football seasons at the New Mexico Military Institute, or NMMI, in Roswell, New Mexico, and then began a huge weight-reduction process to drop to 140 pounds to fight in the lightweight class. Unfortunately, I lost the Golden Gloves championship in the title fights of my two years at NMMI. I thought that my losses to the same fighter were because he was a semiprofessional/professional fighter. And I had only a few weeks to train after the football season ended. Otherwise, I was undefeated in my twenty fights in high school and my junior college fights. In hindsight, maybe I should have pursued a career as a professional boxer. I had the right body. I was talented, as I had a recently retired professional fighter, Charlie McGarity, as my trainer. And I was mentally tough. ***However, going to an academic route sidetracked me, ha!***

During the next twenty years or so—during graduate school, postdoctoral studies, and employment at Warner-Lambert/Parke-Davis, Eastman Pharmaceutics, Isis Pharmaceuticals (now Ionis Pharmaceuticals), NuMax Pharmaceuticals, Biota, and, currently, Carlsbad Pharmaceuticals - I mainly focused on 5Ks, 10Ks, half marathons, marathons, duathlons, and triathlons. My goal was to finish in the top 10 percent of my age group in these cardio events, ***which I never failed to accomplish.***

So much for the early years of my physical fitness endeavors. How do I stack up in my later years? Below, I provide some relative current comparisons.

1. **National physical fitness comparison values for older individuals.** As noted in ***Chapter 2***, I compared myself to my age group and was significantly better in all areas, and even much better than those twenty years younger.
2. **Military physical fitness values based on age.** I did the same comparisons—myself versus the various military branches. I compared well with the younger age groups.

Today at the gym, I was doing triceps press-downs at the cable station. After four sets, each to fatigue, I immediately went to the dip station and did four sets of strict dips. By *strict*, I mean I stayed as upright as possible to focus on my triceps rather than my pecs. A fellow gym guy watched me for both movements. He finally came up and boldly asked me how old I was. When I told him I was seventy-three, he first displayed a shocked look, followed by a look of disappointment. He was disappointed because he was only sixty-two but looked really fit; he was surprised because I looked better than he did, even though I am a lot older.

Another situation happened recently that *"made my day"*. Coming out of Costco, a fellow brassily walked up to me as I was going to my car and noted that I looked good. *My usual response in such situations is to say, "Drugs."* The person usually adopts a sad or shocked expression, and I say I was kidding and move on. But this guy, who was maybe fifty-five or sixty years old, wanted to talk. He asked me about my training program, and so I spent about ten minutes talking to him. Then, I mentioned that I was seventy-three, and he was so much more impressed. What was most interesting about this encounter was that I had not been at the gym beforehand. Actually, I was on the way to 24 Hour Fitness, so I was not pumped at all.

In *Chapter 19 - Pushup Challenge*, I describe an attempt to utilize push-ups to obtain an effective cardiorespiratory event.

BODY MOVEMENTS

Below, I've listed the maximum reps in several body-weight movements and dumbbell lifts I recently accomplished:

* Push-ups: 75, 55, 30
* One-armed push-ups: 20 each
* Parallel dips: 42, 28, 18
* Wide-grip pull-ups: 35, 22,16
* Hammer pull-ups: 40, 28, 19
* Chin-ups (close grip, palms facing body): 36, 22, 17
* Dumbbell bench press, seventy-five pounds: 10, 8, 6
* Dumbbell dead lifts, ninety pounds: 12, 10, 8

HIGHLIGHTS OF MY PHYSICAL FITNESS LIFE AND VARIOUS ASPECTS IMPORTANT TO MY PHYSICAL FITNESS

A number of distinct physical fitness endeavors are related to my lifetime *pursuit of exceptional physical fitness*. I will discuss these separately in the following chapters and later they will be mentioned in various physical fitness programs.

I had already determined that just bag work or push-ups can get my heart rate up to a high level, but doing push-ups or hitting the bag for thirty minutes is tough and boring. But doing these alternately after getting my heart rate up to a high level from running or biking is an excellent way to go. I will discuss this more in **Part 7**.

Also, I am using elastic bands and tubes in about half of my workouts. I continue to mix barbells, dumbbells, machines, and bands or tubes for my strength training.

I have never been overweight. My weight for the past twenty-five years has been 143 pounds, plus or minus one pound. I do have some health and sports problems, which I describe later.

PART 3

Early Days (Ages Six to Thirty)

Chapter 5 - Beginning Early Physical Fitness Days

MY PARENTS MIGRATED IN THE mid-1930s from Wellington, a small town in West Texas, to a dryland farm in the little highway town of Melrose, New Mexico. (Well, the farm was twelve miles inland from the highway town.) I spent the first thirteen years of my life there. *I strongly believe that those years made me mentally and physically tough.* They would make anybody tough! During my years on the farm, I encountered things that surely provided a basis for my eventual *"pursuit of exceptional physical fitness"*.

My father was an acclaimed athlete in Wellington. This was verified in his many scrapbooks containing published accounts from various newspapers. He was a football player who performed on scholarships at several colleges in the area. But more noteworthy was his boxing career in the West Texas area. He was an accomplished fighter, having won titles as a semipro and early professional fighter.

On our desolate, dry farm, my father had installed a heavy bag and a speed bag for boxing training, as well as other items, such as a pole vault and high jump pits, hurdles, and a baseball diamond. He employed black workers from West Texas who lived in several houses on our farm for several months a year. They worked on the farm and participated on the weekends in various athletic events. *My first experience with exceptional physical activity was seeing one of the workers jump up, grasp a two-by-four rafter in the ceiling, and perform several one-armed pull-ups!* This was an incredible display of strength. I know very well, as I have tried and failed to do this at the gym for years. *I can do many one-armed push-ups, though. Ha!*

In my early years, my father and I were very close; he spent as much time as he could with me, considering the effort required to run the farm. *He pushed me to be first in line, to get the first punch in, and to recognize wrestlers' muscles* - muscles without any definition. Someone with wrestlers' muscles might have big, strong arms but without definition between the biceps, triceps, and deltoids. I must note that at my elderly age of seventy-three, I have considerable definition in my arms, as well as my legs and abs. I did not inherit this—it is a result of my lifetime *pursuit of exceptional physical fitness*, as I will discuss in detail later. Some recent pictures of me at age seventy-three are provided in **Part 13.**

On the farm in the 1940s and 1950s, we did not have a telephone or a television, but we got some radio stations. During my early days on the farm, I would sit with my father and listen to the *Pabst Blue Ribbon Bouts.* My father was intensely interested in the fights, having personally known some of the fighters.

My first physical fitness training with my father occurred was when I was six years old. This started "*my life in pursuit of exceptional physical fitness*". My brother Billy was seven years older, and Daddy had Billy perform *HIIT.* Ha! High-intensity interval training has become, in recent years, the major type of cardio fitness training. This is my current approach to cardio training. And in various ways, I have tried to incorporate this into my strength training programs, as I will discuss later.

My father's approach to *HIIT* for my brother was to have him run from one electrical pole to the next on our farm and then jog to the next pole. Note, I did not say *telephone* poles, as we did not have any type of telephone. In an effort to keep up, I ran as best as I could through all the poles, never stopping. *This cardio work and my heavy bag work, described in Chapter 20, were the beginning of my pursuit of exceptional physical fitness, 67 years ago.*

DOGS

An important part of my being raised on a farm was our dogs. My father acquired a pack of ten retired greyhounds that had been racing at the dog tracks in Juarez, Mexico. My interactions with these dogs and several we already had, had an important impact on my life. *This has led to my book "Our Dogs", which is in progress.* My immediate family—my wife, Connie, and our kids, Jess, Danee, and Kim—are all serious dog lovers, and the book discusses the thirty dogs that have thus far been part of our lives. Currently, Danee (Major Cook, retired from the army) is a supervisor at the Oceanside Humane Society, and Kim is board-certified veterinarian specializing in emergency medicine and a supervisor at a major veterinary hospital in Carlsbad, California. Jess and family live in Taos, New Mexico, and have several sweet pit bulls.

CHAPTER 6 - EARLY INNOVATIONS

SUPPLEMENTS

IN MY EARLY DAYS ON the farm, I somehow became aware of protein supplementation. Maybe this was through some magazines my father had; I likely saw an advertisement for protein supplements for bodybuilding. This was when I was ten years old. Maybe I was influenced by the ad showing a well-built bodybuilder on the beach, kicking sand on an underdeveloped person. While I don't remember the exact ad, I recall the product—a protein powder described as "protein of the sea." So, at an early age, I ordered some of this protein and used it as long as I could round up the cost. I now know that *"protein of the sea"* was simply a powder made from dried fish. It was hard to take in, as it just flowed up from the container as a mist. I searched online for this product and found that a similar product is still available. Yuck!

Leg Weights

Judy, my older sister of two years, and I had various chores around the farm. One of the memorable chores was to milk (by hand) several cows each morning and night. We had to wean the calves off the mother cows' milk by going from four teats to none. I also got to watch my father castrate bulls. We ate the fried testicles later that day! I can go on and on about life on the farm.

Judy was an important contributor to my physical fitness development. From a shooting range nearby, we were able to collect a lot of lead shot. My father was an avid hunter of deer, turkey, and the like. He would always bring back several deer to be butchered for venison to eat during the following year. He also had several of the deer hides tanned and converted into nice leather material. From this, my sister and I constructed leg bands containing the lead shot from the shooting range to fit around my legs. Then, *I wore these during my early workouts. This is rather amazing, considering that these efforts took place between 1955 and 1957.*

Chapter 7 - Junior High and High School

First Strength Training

An interesting event occurred in my ninth-grade year (1959) at East Junior High in Roswell, New Mexico. One on the coaches asked me if I would be willing to come to school early on Monday, Wednesday, and Friday mornings to work with some "new" equipment. He had acquired a barbell and two dumbbells and wanted to try them out. Of course, I happily volunteered. We did *"strength training"* for about half of the school year. This was certainly my introduction to strength training by barbells and dumbbells. I did not come into contact with an assortment of strength training equipment until seventeen years later -1976 - at Wall-to-Wall Nautilus in Ann Arbor, Michigan. So, my initial encounter with this coach was foresighted.

As I mentioned earlier, I was the quarterback on the football team and the starting point guard in basketball. I also ran distances in track. I was voted the outstanding athlete for 1959 at East Junior High.

MAKING WEIGHT

Moving on to high school in Roswell, I participated in football, basketball, track, and boxing. I was not a large athlete - five feet eight and 140 to 165 pounds. As noted, for football, I pushed my weight up to 165 and then dropped down to 140 for boxing in the lightweight class. This was surely an interesting dietary accomplishment for a high school and college athlete back in those early days.

We moved to Roswell to from Fort Sumner, New Mexico, in 1957. In the summer of 1963, my father was in the carpenters' union, and I was in the labor union, and we often worked on the same jobs. There was a time I was desperately trying to lose weight for a coming boxing weigh-in; I wanted to make the 140-pound class. After not eating and drinking for two days before the weigh-in, I was weak. When nobody was looking, Daddy would grab a sledgehammer or another tool and do my job, as well as his.

Things didn't always go so smoothly between us. For instance, my father was somewhat upset when I knocked holes in the garage to hang my heavy bag. He thought that a much neater way would have been possible through the attic.

On another occasion, in a high school basketball game, I thought the opposing center aggressively fouled me, so I whacked him in the face with a powerful straight right. Yes, of course, I was kicked out of the game, which was nearly unheard of in high school sports. Daddy was so upset that he could not talk to me about it, but he wrote me a letter letting me know how disappointed he was.

In high school, from tenth grade to twelfth grade, I played football and basketball, ran distances in track, and boxed. In football, I played quarterback and wide receiver, returned kickoffs and punts, and played defensive safety. I was the starting point guard in basketball. As noted above, our mile medley team, which I anchored by running the half-mile leg, beat the state record several times in 1962. I was undefeated in my boxing efforts. I was voted the outstanding athlete of Roswell High School for 1962.

DUNKING

I performed an interesting ***physical fitness endeavor*** in my senior year of high school. This was a period when dunking a basketball became quite important in the NBA, both for the players and for the audience. Well, I certainly could not dunk a basketball at five foot eight, but maybe I could dunk something else. To dunk a basketball, you need to be able to "palm," or grip, the basketball and jump high enough to get your wrist over the rim and slam the ball down. Although I could not get my wrist above the rim, I could get several fingers above it. So, this is what I did: I got a tennis ball (which I could hold in the tips of my fingers), took the shoe off my right foot (the one you pull up on your jump, to lighten the load), and managed to "dunk" a tennis ball. ***Yo-ho!*** This is a good example of my early desire to excel in physical activities.

WATER PADDLES

In the early days of ***Muhammad Ali (Cassius Clay),*** one of my all-time heroes, an issue of *Sports Illustrated* reported that he would perform shadowboxing in a swimming pool. The water would be about neck high, and he would use the water as resistance to his punches. This was quite innovative for the time. In a takeoff of this, a few years later, I decided to glue plywood paddles to the bottom of my Chuck Taylor high-top tennis shoes. I would run in place in the swimming pool, with the water between waist high and chest high. This provided an excellent cardio workout with little stress on my knees. *I think I should have filed a patent on this idea.*

CHAPTER 8 - JR. COLLEGE DAYS – NMMI 1963-1964

MY ATHLETIC EFFORTS AT ROSWELL High School resulted in my receiving a football scholarship to the New Mexico Military Institute, a junior college in Roswell. There, I was a starting running back, played some wide receiver, was the safety, and returned punts and kickoffs. In those days, football players typically played both ways. It's worth mentioning that Roger Staubach began his college athletic career at the New Mexico Military Institute two years before I attended. As we know, he subsequently attended the Naval Academy and won the 1963 Heisman Trophy, spent four years in the US Navy - including a tour of duty in Vietnam - and then came back and eventually won two Super Bowls with the Dallas Cowboys. He is in the Football Hall of Fame.

A life-changing event happened in my second year of football at NMMI. On the day before our Thanksgiving game in 1964, I was hit on the outside of my left knee. In those days, there was scant information on how to treat such injuries. My treatment was to immobilize my left leg by placing a cast from my ankle to my crotch for several weeks. I was able to do push-ups and pull-ups while I recovered, but upon getting out of the cast, my leg was nothing but skin and bones. I had lost most muscle mass.

After graduating from NMMI with an associate's degree, I enrolled in Eastern New Mexico University (ENMU) in Portales, New Mexico. *There began my interest in science as a vocation, which would last for fifty-two years.* I still was not finished with football, as I was a walk-on for the ENMU football team, but my quickness was severely compromised from my knee injury. And quickness and other talents were essential for me to be an effective football player. So, football, which I had excelled at for six years, was gone. However, I could still run distances, bike, and box. Also, I do believe that I could have made the ENMU basketball team.

After the football seasons at NMMI, I began my boxing efforts. I formed and managed a boxing club and was its primary fighter. For my two years at NMMI, I was able to work closely with young high school and junior college cadets, teaching them to step up and be tough.

As noted in **Chapter 4**, in the two years at NMMI, although I was not able to fight until the football season was over, I was undefeated in all my subsequent fights, except for the 1963 and 1964 Golden Gloves championships. There, fighting in the open division, I met up with the same semiprofessional fighter for two years and lost decisions on both fights. ***Thinking back on this situation, I was not mentally ready to get the job done.***

My father offered to pay my college costs when I enrolled in Eastern New Mexico University if I continued my boxing career. This would require me to travel to Clovis, about twenty miles from Portales, for training six days a week. The fight club there ***was eager to have me. However, I had just made a very important decision in my life, that it was now time to pursue my science career.***

CHAPTER 9 - COLLEGE YEARS (1965–1973) AND EARLY WORK YEARS (1974–1998)

IN THE LATE 1970S, IN the cities along the coast in Southern California, biking, duathlons, and triathlons were becoming popular, so I bought my first road bike and began to enter biking events and duathlons (biking and running). I did not enter any triathlons at this time, as I was a terrible swimmer. Soon, cardio training and competition, in the forms of running and riding, became my pastime after long hours at work. Back then, I was not concerned with how to do it or the best way to enhance my cardio training.

Later, I began to enter triathlons. I typically was one of the last competitors to exit the water in these events, but I was competitive in the subsequent biking and running legs. Back in the old days on the farm, we did not have swimming pools—we had irrigation ditches and horse tanks!

I did take a session of Masters swimming lessons in Ann Arbor in 1977, which I hoped would help me in triathlons. For some reason, I could never get my body to flatten out in the crawl stroke, and thus my lower body dragged.

Upon moving to Ann Arbor in 1976, I found and joined my first gym, Wall-to-Wall Nautilus. There, I got my first real exposure to Nautilus and other weight machines. But, still, I did not take any training sessions on how to best use and train on this equipment. I also became pretty good at racquetball, which is an in-your-face competitive sport.

I ran my first marathon in 1977 (at the age of thirty-three) in Detroit. Without much knowledge or training, I was able to register a time of three hours and thirty minutes, which I was happy with. At work at Warner-Lambert/ Parke-Davis, I organized and played on a men's basketball team, which competed well in an organized men's league. I also organized a company 5K run. So, I kept quite fit without focusing on precise cardio or strength training techniques.

After spending several years in Rochester, New York, and Great Valley (near Philadelphia) with a start-up drug-discovery company—Eastman Pharmaceutics of which I was a cofounder—I moved to Carlsbad, California, where I was a cofounder of Isis Pharmaceuticals (now Ionis Pharmaceuticals). In Rochester and Great Valley, I found several fitness clubs with all types of equipment.

CHAPTER 10 - TRANSITION INTO FOCUSED PHYSICAL FITNESS TRAINING – 1995 AND COUNTING

IN THE TWENTY YEARS UP TO 1995, my physical activities were primarily focused on activities at social gatherings, such as running clubs and competitions.

It would be about twenty years before I would give up deriving my physical fitness efforts from these social gatherings and competitions and ***simply and solely focus on just physical fitness.***

In the area of Carlsbad, California, in 1989, several fitness clubs - such as Frogs, LA Fitness, 24 Hour Fitness, Gold's Gym, and others - were appearing. I was a member of each of these clubs at various times.

Starting in 1990, I joined a spin-cycling class—maybe one of the first in the area—at Frog's Health Club. Spin cycling is an excellent cardio fitness endeavor. However, this was before I became a heart rate enthusiast. I monitored my level of effort in my spin-cycling classes by how I felt afterward; determining how good my workout was by monitoring my average heart rate over a session had not become a method for me yet. Another positive aspect of this exercise is that other people can be involved in the classes, such as Connie, my wife. For several years afterward, I would hook up my road bike for stationary spinning at home.

INTERESTING DISTANT BIKING

In the 1980s, I did centuries (hundred-mile bike rides). These rides were stressful, as I did not have the available time to train for them appropriately. But they were a serious challenge and much fun.

In the mid-1990s, I was interested in biking longer distances, but that was difficult to do with my work schedule. I decided to bike a portion of the family trip from Carlsbad, California, to our farm twelve miles north of Melrose, New Mexico. I would stop our trip in Fort Sumner, New Mexico, and get on my bike and ride the fifty miles to our farm. I did this a number of times.

More difficult were my bike rides from Roswell, New Mexico, to Ruidoso, New Mexico. This was about an eighty-five-mile ride, climbing 3,573 feet to 6,920 feet. I would ride to the Greyhound bus station in Ruidoso and take the bus back to Roswell. This was a difficult ride, which I managed to accomplish on most of my summer trips to Roswell.

Also, while living in Great Valley, Pennsylvania, and working at the newly formed Eastman Pharmaceuticals company, I often bicycled the twenty-five miles to work and back. I also would get in a strength training session in the midafternoon.

PART 4

Overview of My Current Physical Fitness Program

IN THIS SECTION, I PROVIDE an overview of my current physical fitness program. Details of the cardiorespiratory and strength training aspects of my program are discussed in **Part 5, 6, and 7.** My diet, supplements, medications, and record-keeping efforts are discussed in **Parts 8, 9, and 10**.

SEPARATION OF CARDIO AND STRENGTH TRAINING

To be truly fit, you must pursue a balanced program of cardiorespiratory training and strength training. Some experts would also include stretching and balance work. In the past twenty years, in ***my pursuit of exceptional physical fitness***, I have separated my cardio and strength training sessions. This allows me to perform strength training with completely fresh muscles. For example, if I want to exhaust my biceps effectively and completely, I will not do a significant cardio training session just before my strength training session. That would be counterproductive.

A recent study has shown that people gain 20 percent more arm strength by lifting weights *before* a cardio session rather than after.

The CrossFit physical fitness program bills itself as a combination of cardio and strength training, but I think its approach is mainly strength training and little serious cardio training (maybe enough for a 5K run). My son I and disagree and often discuss this.

CARDIO TRAINING: HIGH-INTENSITY INTERVAL TRAINING (*HIIT*)

Most people, even physical fitness nuts like me, do not like to spend a large amount of time working out, as we have other things to do. Also, if a program is time consuming, it is not likely to be followed appropriately.

To complete the best workouts and in a minimal time, I developed a *HIIT program*. Yes, I'm using buzzwords—just keeping up with all the hype. *HIIT* stands for *"high-intensity interval training."* This type of workout was originally termed *fartlek* (which means "speed play" in Swedish) in Europe about fifty years ago. In the United States, in roughly the past fifty years, this was termed *speed play*. When I ran distances in high school track in Roswell, we referred to this training as such. Recall from **Part 3** that my first encounter with this type of cardio workout was in 1950.

The program I developed is designed to be cardio training, which means it works on your cardiorespiratory system (mainly your heart) and is not in any way related to strength training. I don't think *HIIT* works with strength training, but I have tried to develop an effective program that combines cardio and strength training. (**See Part 7.**)

An effective *HIIT* program does not require running five miles or more (my usual run is about three miles) or biking for miles and miles (my usual distance is eight to twelve miles).

HEART RATE MONITORS AND MAXIMUM HEART RATES

An absolutely essential aspect of my cardio training sessions is that they are "managed" by the level of my heart rate as determined by an effective heart rate monitor. Heart rate monitors are discussed in *Chapter 15*.

CARDIO TRAINING SESSIONS

My current cardio workouts are running and biking. I plan these to last about forty-five minutes for running and about sixty minutes for biking. I have a running day, a biking day, and a rest day, and then I repeat.

STRENGTH TRAINING SESSIONS

I do strength training sessions seven times a week at the gym. My current health club is 24 Hour Fitness, where I have been a member for about twenty years. Typically, I do eight to ten movements daily, taking about four minutes per movement, for a strength training session. An example of a movement is a bicep curl or an abdominal crunch. I have designed these sessions over many years, and it takes about thirty-two to forty minutes for me to complete a workout. I do the strength training in the afternoon, or about five to seven hours after a cardio workout. This allows me sufficient time to recover fully from the cardio effort in the morning. It is important to do strength training with fresh muscles, as you want to maximally exhaust a muscle or muscle group. I don't use a heart rate monitor in my strength training sessions, as proper strength training is not a substitute for cardio training.

In **Parts 5 and 6**, I provide a detailed account of my complete physical fitness program.

In **Part 7**, I describe my efforts to combine cardio and strength training.

DIET

My diet is an essential part of my pursuit of exceptional physical fitness, as it should be for everybody. I describe this in **Part 8**.

SUPPLEMENTS

I consider supplements to be essential in my pursuit of exceptional physical fitness as well. I describe the supplements I take in **Part 9**.

RECORD KEEPING

Record keeping is another essential aspect of my pursuit of exceptional physical fitness and is covered in **Part 10**.

TIME SPENT ON MY PHYSICAL FITNESS PROGRAM

My physical fitness program is composed of four or five cardio training sessions (biking and running) and seven strength training sessions each week. These sessions are of high intensity. ***Overall, they amount to a little over an hour a day, or about 5 percent of my twenty-four-hour day.***

PART 5

Cardio Training

CHAPTER 11 - MONITORED CARDIO TRAINING SESSIONS

I HAVE ALWAYS SAID THAT if I could do only one physical fitness movement, *"it would be running—or now maybe fast walking, in my arthritic later years".* Running and other cardio training sessions would be monitored by a *global positioning system (GPS) heart rate monitors.* These are discussed in *Chapter 14.*

> *Planning my cardiorespiratory training around a select heart rate, preferably my maximum, is an essential aspect of my cardio fitness program.*

In 2010, my maximum heart rate was determined to be *165 beats per minute.* I have had this clinically determined several times since. This was accomplished with a standard maximum stress test performed on a treadmill with an EKG, heart monitors, hookups, and the like. A cardiologist was usually overseeing the procedure.

Cardiologists consider a runner's maximum heart rate to be the highest rate (beats per minute) one reaches during a VO_2 (volume of oxygen) maximum test (a ten- to fifteen-minute treadmill test of progressively increasing difficulty). VO_2 max is a measure of the maximum volume of oxygen that an athlete can use, and this directly relates to your maximum heart rate. My last VO_2 test was in 2012, and I tested out as a thirty-nine-year-old. *Ha!—a real ego trip.*

I'm sure there are at least fifteen devised formulas in the literature to determine your maximum heart rate. One of the first, which is still used, is to calculate your maximum heart rate by **subtracting your age from 220.** This formula would suggest that my maximum, at age seventy-three, is **147.** It is thought that any formula that uses age is not very accurate. However, this calculated value of **147** is close to my maximum heart rate as observed in a real-life situation, noted below. The most recent formula that I have seen is **206.9 – (0.67 × age).** This calculates to a maximum rate of **158** for me.

Another way to determine maximum heart rate is to overexert yourself at the end of a run or bike ride. Preferably going up a steep hill, **push hard until you think death is near—as in the next step or pedal.** Then, look at the number on your heart rate monitor. This value will be quite close to your maximum heart rate. **Note that this method should be reserved for experienced athletes!** In considering this, I currently often max out with a run, bike ride, or pull-up session after a run or bike ride at **155** beats per minute.

If I consider the above, my maximum heart rate could be **147, 155, or 158**—all similar.

Any of these calculated values provides a number that you can base your workouts on. By using a selected heart rate value in a cardio workout, you can ask, **"How did I compare to my last cardio session?"** or determine an average over several workouts. Over a few cardio sessions, you can recognize a heart rate number that represents an intense level, and this can become a target for subsequent cardio sessions.

I consider my average heart rate over a running or biking cardio session to be my best measurement for cardiovascular fitness training. In my early years of cardio training, I found that an intense cardio workout for me was about **75 percent to 80 percent of my maximum heart rate of 165 (75 percent of 165 equals 124; 80 percent of 165 equals 132).** I still pursue the 75 percent to 80 percent level, but my maximum heart rate has decreased about a beat to a beat and a half per year, according to scientific studies. Today, I am using **155 beats per minute as my maximum**, as determined above.

In my recent cardio sessions, I have taken to performing an all-out sprint (as best as I can accomplish) in the last one hundred yards of my running sessions or the last quarter mile of my biking sessions. *Maybe I am just trying to kill myself—fall over dead in the ditch, and get it over with!* I typically register a value of about **153** beats per minutes, which is **99 percent of 155.**

Because of my **HIIT** approach, for the past several years, I have pursued the intense portion of my running by going up the incline of hills on streets. This is a great way to get a high heart rate; unfortunately, I have to run/walk back down. I'm in great shape, so my heart rate drops to near average when I do this. This does not result in a high average heart rate for the session.

However, a more serious problem is the actual run-walk back down the incline. Every time I plant my foot for the next step, I am essentially putting the brakes on, and most of my body weight is on my planted foot. This causes a lot of knee pain. Finally, after about sixty-seven years, *I figured out that I should restrict my downhill runs.*

I typically run on a flat surface—the sidewalk, a track, or the pavement. Running on the grass next to the concrete course at the park or other places is easier on my knees. However, I have never liked to run on grass (except maybe in a football game) or dirt, as the surface is soft and uneven.

My most intense cardio workouts are when I ride up a series of the steep hills in Cardiff, California. The most intense is Birmingham Drive, about a half mile from bottom to top and super steep (about a 10 percent incline). A rule of mine is that once I decide to ride up a hill, I never stop or turn around; rather, I go all out to get to the top. I like to stay seated in my bicycle seat, but on most of these hills, I have to stand up for an all-out effort. It is difficult and dangerous to stop or turn around midway up the hill. After all, you must deal with getting your feet out of the clip pedals, face the traffic, and then go down rather than continue up.

I do a particular hill about once a week, usually just before going on a relatively flat eight- to ten-mile course. This helps my final average heart rate. I typically register my highest maximum heart rate on these rides. Yesterday, at age seventy-three, I barely managed to get to the top. This was a day after a heavy leg-strength session, and maybe I hadn't eaten well the day before. Still, my heart rate peaked at *152*. I consider my current maximum heart rate to be *155*. Thus, on this climb, I got up to 98 percent of my max. I think this is impressive, and it did affect the rest of my ride, as my average heart rate was *130*, or *84 percent*.

I take 400 mg of Advil about an hour before a cardio workout session and wear Ace elastic knee supports for my runs. These are too tight for biking. Recently, I started taking two Aleve tablets along with Advil before my cardio workouts. These painkillers work nicely for me. If I don't take them before my running cardio sessions, my knee pain prevents me from having an effective session.

On being asked, *"How did your cardio session go?"* I usually respond with, *"I am near death."* Recently, I have begun to think there is considerable truth to this. But then I look at my Garmin to see my average heart rate from the session and how well I did.

Fortunately or unfortunately, I do tend to continue to increase the intensity of my cardio sessions as I age. I mentioned earlier that as I've aged, I have increased my physical fitness efforts, unlike others my age. How long can I continue to do this?

CHAPTER *12* - CURRENT CARDIO WORKOUT

AS I NOTED, I USE *speed play* for my running cardio sessions—meaning fast walking, jogging, or running—until I am winded to some extent or for a set period, such as thirty seconds. I reduce my pace to a walk or slow jog to recover, and then I repeat the process. I continue to do this at a pace of about fifteen minutes per mile for two to three miles, for a total of thirty to forty-five minutes. I apply this approach to my biking sessions as well. These are a bit longer at approximately sixty minutes at ten to twelve miles per hour. The purpose of the **HIIT** approach is to elevate my heart rate to a high level throughout the workout. I consider a high level of heart rate for a significant time to be a *"training effect"*.

I want to average *75 percent to 80 percent of my maximum heart rate (75 percent to 80 percent of 155, or 116 to 124)*, so these are *intense workouts*, but they last only forty-five to sixty minutes. Of course, essential for my cardio sessions is a heart rate monitor so I can know my final average and check during my run or ride to make adjustments to my speed. Heart rate monitors are discussed in **Chapter 14.**

At the beginning of my cardio workouts, I do a set of push-ups (about fifty), sit-ups (about twenty-five), and pull-ups (about twenty-five). I do these before *every* cardio run or bike ride. At the end of my run or ride, I do a set of heavy-bag work (about three minutes), push-ups (about forty), sit-ups (about twenty), and pull-ups (about twenty-five), taking a total of about ten minutes. This portion of my cardio workout actually raises my heart rate. Also, I have found that in the last movement, the pull-ups, *I typically achieve a high heart rate of 152 beats per minute, which is about 98 percent of my maximum.*

To summarize, each cardio session is forty-five to sixty minutes of running or biking with about ten minutes of pre- and post workout movements at an average heart rate of 75 percent to 80 percent of my max. This is extremely aggressive!

If my workout does not provide a high average heart rate, then I not only have wasted an hour but also (and maybe more important) have stressed my body for no benefit.

I typically plan my cardio sessions for Monday, Wednesday, and Friday, or twelve times a month. In the past year, to increase my cardio training, I have introduced two cardio sessions back to back, followed by a rest day. This provides twenty days of cardio training a month. For example, I bike one day, run the next day, rest the next, and repeat the sequence. My back-to-back cardio workouts are bike/run/rest, run/bike/rest, or bike/bike/rest. I never do a run/run/rest (back-to-back runs). I have found that my knees do not support this type of doubling up.

I complete my cardio sessions early enough, by nine thirty in the morning, so that I have about six hours of rest before my strength training sessions.

Training partners are vital. *"Honey Pearl"*, one of our three pugs, is one of my favorite training partners. She gives me kisses when I do my push-ups. Another favorite pug is *"Harley-Man"*; he likes to get on my body as I do sit-ups. *I can't imagine life without at least two dogs, particularly pugs.*

One of the most enjoyable parts of running or walking in the neighborhood is meeting and talking to the dogs that people are walking. On a typical run, I meet up with about five dogs. I ask the owners if I can talk to their dogs, and everybody happily agrees. This brief time fits nicely into my **HIIT** cardio session.

In a recent duathlon—5K run, 20K bike, and 5K run—my daughters ran the first and last legs, and I biked the middle leg, which was a 20K ride (12.4 miles). My plan was to try to average at least **80 percent (124 beats per minute)** of my maximum, as in training. To my great surprise, I averaged **141 beats per minute, or 91 percent of my maximum**. Being pushed in competition certainly resulted in a greater output. *"You never know everything"*.

CHAPTER 13 - HEAVY LEG-STRENGTH TRAINING FOR RUNNING

As NOTED, I HAVE KNEE problems, particularly in my left knee, the one I injured playing football in 1964. Arthritis has also been an issue for the past ten years and is getting worse. Not only is there pain in walking and running, but also *I have become significantly bowlegged. I was five foot eight for years, but in the past twenty years, my height has declined to about five foot six.* More important, in the past year, it has been painful for me to run or speed walk fast enough to achieve significant cardio training. I have always thought that if I cannot get a significant cardio session in, I am just torturing myself and should not continue this workout program. Because of my progressing knee problems, I quit doing any type of strength training for my legs in the past year.

But after reading various articles concerning arthritis, it became clear that simply quitting any kind of legwork or weight-bearing exercise was not the way to go. In fact, a recent study found *a 43 percent reduction in knee pain in subjects who participated in lower-body weight training, such as squats.*

So, I recently reintroduced the complete leg workout I routinely did in previous years. Details of my high-intensity leg workouts are described in **Part 6**.

To my amazement, I experienced greatly reduced pain during my running workouts and was able to complete all my running cardio sessions. *So, heavy leg workouts and running* do *go together, certainly for me.*

Also, a recent study suggests that runners don't suffer more long-term damage to their knee joints compared with nonrunners. The study of more than 2,600 middle-aged participants found *that people who ran more actually experienced* **less** *knee pain over time.* The study examined medical data from people whose average age was sixty-four. Researchers set out to examine both regular knee pain and pain associated with arthritis. They discovered a surprising trend: *the more people had run in their lives, the less knee pain they felt at the time of the survey.* In fact, only about 21 percent of people who ran regularly also reported having knee pain, compared with about 25.3 percent of former runners and 29.6 percent of people who had never run for exercise.

The study's evidence aligns with previous research that has found running to have no effect on the development of cumulative joint pain and arthritis. Research also indicates that running is associated with a host of health benefits, from less stress and better memory to lower cancer risk and even a longer life.

I must note that I'm not at all sure of the results of these studies. My knee problems have gradually gotten worse over the past twenty years and continue today. But my heavy leg-strength training has definitely helped my running, and I will certainly continue it.

CHAPTER 14 - HEART RATE MONITORS

I COULD NOT IMAGINE LIFE without a heart rate monitor! In other words, as a physical fitness nut that requires considerable cardio training, a heart rate monitor is *absolutely essential, and specifically, a heart rate monitor that has a global positioning system (GPS).*

My monitor tells me what my average heart rate is over a workout period and how it compares with my maximum heart rate. If you do speed play for the same distance or course every other day and time it with your watch, you will know how long the workout took on a particular day, *but you will not know how hard you worked your heart!*

You can say, *"Oh, I really worked hard today! I'm even sweating somewhat!"* and use various other perceived factors, but this will not directly relate to your heart's activity. My son and I often discuss the aspects of perceived effort, as he is not entirely into heart rate monitors. I usually end the discussion by noting that he could just sit on the couch, have a beer, and perceive that he got a meaningful workout. Ha!

I should note that with the *"speed-play approach"*, you can pick a course and essentially do the same thing every workout. For many, *this is good - at least you are doing something* - but I think you should try to increase the intensity of your workouts reasonably. **This can be accurately determined only by monitoring your average heart rate over the workout session.**

I love my current monitor. It does a lot of things, even though most of them aren't necessary. I bought some of the first types of Polar heart rate monitors ever marketed, more than twenty years ago, and have been using some type ever since. The early heart rate monitors did not have the GPS function; in fact, many of the current heart rate monitors still do not have this.

My current monitor is a Garmin Forerunner 405 CX (GPS). I first bought this model about ten years ago. It was $300 and came with a heart rate strap and a wireless connection to my computer.

I do my workout and walk into my office (*within fifteen feet of my computer*). Within a minute or two, the workout data is wirelessly downloaded to my computer. Cool! The data is saved and can be graphed in several ways. The monitor also records about fifty other things, including time of workout, heart rate, average heart rate, heart rate versus time/distance/elevation gain, percent grade, temperature, wind factor, virtual training, warning of turns, and the point of returning from an out-and-back run or ride. *Most impressive, it records the precise distance you moved (GPS).*

This is also a wristwatch monitor that I wear daily. One of these may impress your coworkers! Any effective heart rate monitor must have a heart rate strap that you put around your chest before you go for your speed play. Monitors that require you only to touch the face of your watch to get an instantaneous reading will not get the job done because they do not provide an average heart rate over a workout session. Similarly, monitors that use a strap but give only an instantaneous reading will not provide the average heart rate over the session.

The model I have has been out of production for five years, but some companies are still selling watches on Amazon, now for about $150. I did buy one of these as an eventual backup, but it did not work, and I had to return it. Newer models of my current Garmin are available. They have a touch screen and come in various colors for about $350 to $500. But for me, these have too many unnecessary functions.

So, the question is, what type of heart rate monitor should I invest in? *A heart rate monitor that will record my current time, distance, and heart rate and final time, distance, and average heart rate over the workout session would cost about $150.* The big difference here is that this less expensive model does not record distance.

I dearly hope that I can find an effective replacement when my current monitor wears out. Looking at the current literature on available Garmin monitors, I see several Garmin watches that appear to do everything I require (and, of course, many other things). One records your heart rate from your wrist rather than from a chest band. I read some time ago that heart rate measurement from the wrist is not as accurate as from the chest. Upon further study, I found that this Garmin watch does not provide the average heart rate over the training session.

CHAPTER 15 - BICYCLES

OBVIOUSLY, ONE NEEDS A BIKE for biking cardio training sessions. After much consideration, several years ago, I brought a *Litespeed Ghisallo Titanium bike for $8,000.* Yes, it is the fourth-most expensive thing I have ever bought, after a house, car and college cost for our kids. But I was and am serious about my physical fitness and wanted a high-level bike that would take the question *"How good is my bike?"* out of the equation. This purchase certainly accomplished this. I have replaced the tires a few times and have kept everything adjusted and lubricated.

I am so happy, lucky that I realized the value of serious biking relatively early in my physical fitness endeavors! I can use this cardio training method for the rest of my life. I do support my biking efforts with strength training movements, such as knee lifts, backward kicks, and other leg movements, discussed in **Part 6**.

CHAPTER *16* - E-BIKES AND TREADMILLS

I HAVE NOTED THAT IF I could do only one cardio training event, it would be running. Of course, biking would be next. Believe it or not, Southern California does have some days of bad weather. They are rare, but I don't like to run or ride on rainy, cold days, and I don't like to miss a cardio workout session. On such days, I can accomplish a good cardio running session on a treadmill at my health club. In fact, there is a huge advantage for me to run on a treadmill in that it offers level running or inclined running with no downhills (declines), which, as I have noted, are difficult for me. The treadmills at my health club are amazing. They have a lever to increase or decrease the speed and a lever to increase or decrease the incline. One's percent incline, speed (miles per hour), average speed for a workout, current time spent, and current heart rate are displayed on the front of the treadmill. The most important readout, I think, is the average heart rate over the cardio session. This is not provided, but I wear my Garmin monitor, which provides this and my maximum heart rate. I am not ready to completely give up running outside for a club treadmill. But some days, it is certainly a reasonable replacement.

I have found that occasional cardio biking workouts on a club e-bike (rather than biking outside) are not so good. Currently, I use high-intensity interval training (***HIIT***) for all my cardio training sessions. For outside biking, my portion of ***HIIT*** is biking up 250- to 300-yard hills of about 10 percent inclines. In my usual eight- to ten-mile bike ride, I get in about thirteen of these climbs. These are so intense that I typically register a heart rate close to my maximum, but I have not been able to replicate this on an e-bike. I could not increase my revolutions or intensity enough to come anywhere close to my maximum heart rate. My average heart rate on an e-bike is about 115 beats per minute (74 percent) compared with 130 beats per minute (84 percent) biking outside. But there are some advantages of using an e-bike rather than outside biking, certainly considering the weather.

PART 6

Strength Training

A RECENT STUDY FOUND THAT strength training as you age reduces your risk for death. Researchers surveyed people aged sixty-five or older about their exercise habits and then tracked them for fifteen years. Nearly one-third of the study participants died during that period. Under 10 percent of the subjects engaged in strength training, but those select few were 46 percent less likely to die during the study.

In my strength training sessions, I typically utilize the standard barbells, dumbbells, and weight machines that are found in health clubs, as well as the elastic materials I bring with me, for the latter aren't generally found in health clubs. I also use body-weight movements.

CHAPTER 17 - STRENGTH TRAINING WITH ELASTIC MATERIALS - BANDS/TUBES

ELASTIC MATERIALS (BANDS AND TUBES) have played a major role in my strength training workouts for about ten years. Interestingly, I have been going to health clubs for forty years, and rarely do I see the attendees using elastic materials. For sure, the clubs do not furnish these materials, mainly because such workouts do not require a health club. You can easily carry out these workouts in a garage or living room and thus not have to pay a club membership fee. However, my strength training sessions involve a combination of the equipment found at clubs and elastic materials, so I do regularly attend a 24 Hour Fitness club. Also, I believe in *"misery likes company"* so there is a much better chance that I will get my complete workouts in, if I go to a strength training club.

Elastic materials allow you to perform resistive exercises. The materials come in different thickness levels to allow you to change the resistance for a particular exercise and to accommodate users with varying levels of strength. The thickness of the band or tube and the place where you grip it to change its length determine its resistance level.

With typical weight movements (using dumbbells, barbells, cables, and so on), the intensity (resistance) does not increase over the positive contraction movement (such as raising the dumbbell in a curl). In the case of bands and tubes, however, the intensity increases with the length of the movement. For example, if you are doing a bicep curl with a twenty-five-pound dumbbell, the exercise actually gets easier as your forearm and the dumbbell get farther above a parallel line to the floor. This is because your elbow is assisting in the exercise. With elastic materials, the resistance *increases* as the band or tube is stretched, offsetting the leverage of your elbow. Another, maybe more important, advantage that you can gain with bands and tubes is that you can introduce *power movements - rapid movements against resistance, such as jumping, pitching a baseball, and throwing a punch (important, yes!)*. All these are functional movements, meaning that they relate to real-life movements instead of, say, doing a bicep curl.

There are some differences between bands and tubes. Tubes typically come with handles. Of course, you can grip the tube and not use the handles, but this is not comfortable. Bands, on the other hand, typically do not have handles, but handles can be attached. With bands, you can easily grip anywhere on the band and monitor the resistance, which is a much easier way to go, as I have found. But in a *complete strength training session*, you would need to use both bands and tubes. Both can be of various levels of thickness and width to provide various levels of initial resistance.

Bands provide a much smoother exercise through the entire range of motion. Often, people working out at the gym will rapidly push a weight up and then aggressively stop it on the way down. Elastic materials kill momentum, making them excellent for strength training and muscle building. Training with elastic materials allows you to move explosively without the fear of flying weights, making them an excellent choice for power training.

Another advantage to using elastic materials for training instead of free weights or machines is that the materials are portable. They are light enough to carry to the gym in a small bag.

I bring to the gym a small bag that contains a high-resistance tube with handles, a thin high-resistance band (four inches wide and six feet long), and a six-foot circular band (a quarter of an inch thick and two inches wide). The total cost for these elastic materials is under fifty dollars.

How many of my strength movements can be effectively accomplished with elastic bands or tubes? I have developed effective movements with elastic materials for every movement I want to do. Leg exercises such as squats, dead lifts, and calf raises are easy to do with them.

CHAPTER 18 - STRENGTH TRAINING MOVEMENTS

STRENGTH TRAINING RELATES TO THE whole body, which I describe in three overlapping parts: legs, core, and upper body.

I divide my strength training sessions into seven days each week; primarily, I focus on a specific body part each day. Thus, my program involves triceps, shoulders, biceps, and the chest. For the past year, I have gone back to doing heavy legwork every fourth day. I also do at least one core movement every day. The first three days are mainly isolated movements (focused on a single joint). But absolute single-joint movements are difficult to achieve. The push-and-pull days involve compound movements. These primarily work a specific muscle group but with support from other muscles—typically those that were isolated in the first three days. This addresses the concern that you need to work each muscle group more than once a week.

I try to get in eight to ten movements in each workout and sometimes as many as twelve. I do three or four sets for each movement (around five to twelve repetitions), each to fatigue. The total time for a movement is about four minutes. This includes setting up the desired weight and moving between stations. *I work fast!*

At this rate, each of my strength training sessions lasts from thirty-two to forty minutes. This means I can exert maximal effort for each muscle group, as is the proper method. I do about seventy movements over seven days for my strength training work. This amounts to about four hours a week for strength training. Some people may consider my strength training sessions to be just bodybuilding, as *Arnold Schwarzenegger may have done. That may be so, but I also do extensive cardio sessions; I carefully separate the two.* My time in cardio training—four to five days at about fifty minutes per day—is about four hours a week. *So, in total, I currently invest a little more than sixty minutes a day for my physical fitness efforts.*

I list the strength training movements and core movements that I typically perform in my seven days of strength training. One will note that free weights, cable/weight machines, elastic bands/tubes and body weight are employed. I identify *Weight Machines* as equipment that one adds plates (weights) to provide the desired resistances. *Cable Machines* are equipment that one adjusts the resistance by insertion of a pin into a rack of weights. Of course *dumbbells and barbells* are weights with various attached weight plates. The cables of *Cable Machines* are typically attached to handles.

I note where elastic materials are used, and of these, the ones I believe that are superior movements to weight and cable machine movements, and likely novel.

MONDAY – Triceps/Core

1. **Parallel dips**
   - *2.1.* This is a compound body movement, but I lean my upper body back to focus on my triceps as much as possible. Obviously, pectorals, laterals, and chest muscle groups will be worked.
     - *1.1.1.* My usual effort is three sets to fatigue (typically, about forty, twenty-five, and fifteen reps).
   - *1.2.* To provide more resistance and reduce the number of reps, I often hang a ten- or twenty-five-pound plate from my hips with my circular band.
2. **Seated cable-machine triceps press-downs**
   - *2.1.* I usually do six sets to fatigue, reducing the weight for the fourth, fifth, and six sets.
3. **Standing triceps press-downs with bands**
   - *3.1.* Using my thin band doubled and wrapped around and behind my neck, I do six sets to fatigue, reducing the resistance for the fourth, fifth, and six sets by changing hand positions.
     - *3.1.1.* This is a novel movement. I have never seen anybody do this at the gym.
   - *3.2.* I also attach my thin band to a hook on the triceps press-down cable machine and do sets, changing my grip to change the resistance.
4. **Band triceps extension lying on bench with band wrapped around my back (typically known as a "skull crusher" when using a barbell)**
   - *4.1.* I do three sets to fatigue, adjusting my handgrip to perform about eight to ten reps per set.

> ***4.1.1. This is a novel movement with the elastic band and much better than the skull crusher with a barbell. I have never seen anybody do this at the gym.***

5. **Standing overhead triceps extensions with an elastic tube**
   - **5.1.** The elastic tube is wrapped around a rail on a cable machine about six or seven feet from the floor. With my back to the support, I grip the handles of the tube over my head and extend my arms.
     - **5.1.1.** I do three sets to fatigue, adjusting my handgrip on the tube to perform about eight to ten reps per set.
       - **5.1.1.1** In this exercise, you can adjust your grip on the handles (e.g., hammerhead, palms up, or palms down).
   - **5.2.** This is often done in the gym with cable machines, ***but using the elastic tube is easier and more effective***

6. **Standing overhead triceps extensions with an elastic tube**
   - **6.1.** The elastic tube is wrapped around a rail on a cable machine about six or seven feet from the floor. With my back to the support, I grip the handles of the tube over my head and extend my arms.
     - **6.1.1.** I do three sets to fatigue, adjusting my handgrip on the tube to perform about eight to ten reps per set.
       - **6.1.1.1** In this exercise, you can adjust your grip on the handles (e.g., hammerhead, palms up, or palms down).
   - **6.2.** This is often done in the gym with cable machines, but using the elastic tube is easier and more effective.

7. **Seated triceps push-downs on cable pec fly machine**
   - **7.1.** This cable machine is different from the one used in number 2. I do three sets to fatigue.
   - **7.2.** *This is a novel movement. I have never seen anybody do this at the gym.*

8. **Close-grip push-ups**
   - **8.1.** This is a compound movement, but the major focus is on the triceps.
     - **8.1.1.** Forefingers and thumbs should be touching in this exercise. I do three sets to fatigue.

8.1.1.1 I typically get in twenty-five reps in the first set. Note that this is the last movement of my triceps workout.

8.1.2. On occasion, I perform dips with my hands placed back on a bench, my legs and feet extending on another bench, and my quadriceps supporting a forty-five-pound plate.

8.1.2.1 This focuses much more on my triceps than the parallel dips described above.

9. **Back extension on incline bench (for the core)**

   9.1. I use my circular band, doubled for resistance, attached to a forty-five-pound plate.

      9.1.1. I do three or four sets.

         9.1.1.1 You can also do this on cable machines at some clubs.

TUESDAY – SHOULDERS/CORE

10. **Standing barbell pull-up or cable-machine pull-up**

   10.1. This is a compound movement. I do three sets to fatigue.

      10.1.1. This exercise works the posterior, lateral, and arterial deltoids.

11. **Seated cable presses or dumbbell presses or band presses (Arnold presses)**

   11.1. To do this with bands, you should be seated with the band under your body. I start with my arms folded in front of my chest and my palms facing my chest, and I end up with my hands above my head and my palms facing away from my body.

      11.1.1. This is a compound movement. I do three sets to fatigue.

   11.2. This works the lateral, anterior, and posterior deltoids.

      11.2.1. This can be done with dumbbells or cables.

> ***11.3. With bands, this is a novel movement. I have never seen anybody do this at the gym.***

12. Repeat 8 and 9 to further exhaust your anterior and lateral deltoids (with some effect on the posterior deltoid).

13. Seated lateral rises

> **13.1.** This is an isolated movement (focused on lateral deltoids).
>> **13.1.1.** This can be done with dumbbells or bands.
> **13.2.** I do three sets to fatigue.

14. Standing front rises (for anterior deltoids)

> **14.1.** These can be done with dumbbells or bands.
>> **14.1.1.** I do three sets to fatigue.

15. Posterior raises (for posterior deltoids)

> **15.1.** Bend over, and place your head on the bench.
>> **15.1.1.** These are done with dumbbells.
> **15.2.** I do three sets to fatigue.

All these shoulder (deltoid) movements can be readily performed with dumbbells, cable machines, or elastic bands. I typically alternate my shoulder workouts with free weights, cable machines, and elastic materials. Use of bands for all the shoulder movements is particularly effective. These movements are much easier to accomplish with bands than with weights or cable machines.

16. **Lateral oblique twists with elastic tube attached to pole (for core)**

> **16.1.** Holding the handles on the tube in front of my body, I rapidly twist my trunk as far to the right as possible and then all the way to the left, moving as rapidly as possible. Resistance is adjusted by moving closer to or away from the pole.
> **16.2.** This is effective core movement, much superior to the version using cable machines that is typically done at clubs.
>> ***16.2.1. This is a novel movement. I have never seen anybody do this at the gym.***

WEDNESDAY – BICEPS/CORE

17. Chin-ups, close grip, palms facing body with two inches between palms

17.1. This is a combination move, but it mainly works the biceps.

17.2. My usual effort is three sets to fatigue, typically about thirty, seventeen, and ten reps.

18. Dumbbell curls on incline bench, palms facing up

18.1. This is an isolated movement.

18.2. I do three sets to fatigue.

19. Standing hammerhead/twist dumbbell curls, alternating arms

19.1. I start with my palms facing the side of my body and end with my palms facing the front of my body.

19.2. I do one set with as many reps as possible, using extensive cheating, to fatigue.

20. Standing barbell drag lift (not a curl)

20.1. Holding the bar with both hands, I raise it in front of my body in a straight line from my waist by pulling my arms back and leaning backward as I lift. I allow the bar to twist in my hands as I lift it. I do three sets to fatigue.

> ***20.1.1. This is an excellent bicep movement, one that I have never seen used in the gym.***

21. Standing hammerhead/twist curls with elastic tubes

21.1. These are rapid movements. I do three sets to fatigue.

21.2. Next, I adjust the resistance by changing the tube length under my foot;
Movements are still rapid. Again, I do three sets to fatigue.

21.3. You can use bands rather than the tube to allow easier adjustment of resistance.

22. Standing reverse curls with elastic bands

22.1. Hands should be facing the body. You can adjust the resistance by changing positioning of the hands. These are rapid movements. I do three sets to fatigue.

23. Handgrip curls

23.1. I adjust the resistance by changing the position of the tube under my foot.

24. Cable-machine crunches (for core)

24.1. I use straight-down crunches mixed with side (oblique) crunches and do three or four sets to fatigue.

THURSDAY – *PUSH/CHEST/CORE*

25. Dumbbell bench presses

25.1. I do four to six sets to fatigue.

25.1.1. I currently start with seventy-five pounds for the first set (about eight reps) and decrease the weight to fifty-five pounds over the remaining sets.

26. Decline presses, weight machine

26.1. I do three or four sets to fatigue.

27. Inclined presses, weight machine

27.1. I do three or four sets to fatigue.

28. Seated Pec fly, cable machine

28.1. I do three or four sets to fatigue.

29. Seated Pec fly, cable machine—press-downs as in parallel dip

29.1. I do three or four sets to fatigue.

30. Seated push-ups twist, cable machine

30.1. I do three or four sets to fatigue.

30.1.1. This can be done with elastic bands on a bench—a novel movement.

31. Hanging leg raises (for core)

FRIDAY – *PULLS/CORE*

32. Pull-ups - palms facing away from body, six inches outside shoulder width

32.1. This is a combination move, but it mainly works the shoulders, lats, and biceps.

    32.1.1. My usual effort is three sets to fatigue, typically about twenty-five, fifteen, and ten reps.

32.1.2. Distance between hands can be adjusted.

33. Inclined pull-downs (high rows), weight machine

    33.1. This is a combination move, but it mainly works the shoulders, lats, and biceps.

    33.2. I do three or four sets to fatigue.

34. Declined pull-ups (low rows), weight machine

    34.1. This is a combination move, but it mainly works the shoulders, lats, and biceps.

    34.2. I do three or four sets to fatigue.

35. Shrug pull-ups, weight machine

    35.1. I do three or four sets to fatigue.

36. Wide-grip lats pull-downs, cable machine

    36.1. I do three or four sets to fatigue.

37. Wide-grip behind-the-neck lats pull-downs, cable machine

    37.1. I do three or four sets to fatigue.

38. Side lifts for obliques (for core)

    38.1. You can grip weight plates; it is better to use bands.

LEGS/CORE – EVERY FOURTH DAY (REPLACE USUAL BODY PART

39. Leg press, cable machine

    39.1. Adjust weight to allow a complete squat.

    39.2. I do four or five sets to fatigue.

40. Dumbbell dead lifts

    40.1. I begin with eighty-five pounds and reduce the weight for the second and third sets.

41. Single leg press, cable machine

    41.1. Adjust the weight to allow a complete squat.

41.2. I do four or five sets to fatigue, alternating between my left leg and my right leg.

42. Leg extension, cable machine

42.1. I do four or five sets to fatigue.

43. Single leg extension, cable machine

43.1. I do four or five sets to fatigue, alternating between my left leg and my right leg.

44. Leg curl, cable machine

44.1. I do four or five sets to fatigue.

45. Single leg curl, cable machine

45.1. I do four or five sets to fatigue, alternating between my left leg and my right leg.

46. Calf raises, cable or weight machine (standing or seated)

46.1. I do four or five sets to fatigue.

47. Reverse calf raises, seated cable machine

47.1. I do four or five sets to fatigue.

48. Knee lifts and backward kicks, elastic band

48.1. Place the circular band on the rack where various handles for cable machines are stored. Do single knee lifts, and alternate with backward kicks.

48.2. I do four or five sets to fatigue.

48.2.1. These can be done on weight machines.

Core Movements

Five movements are required to work the core effectively. I try to do at least one core movement in each strength training session. These movements can be accomplished in numerous ways. The core movements I currently use are noted above and listed below.

1. **Back extension on incline bench**

1.1. I use a circular band, doubled for resistance, and do three or four sets.

1.1.1. This can also be done on some weight machines at some clubs.

2. **Lateral oblique twists with elastic tube attached to pole**
   2.1. Holding the handles on the tube in front of my body, I rapidly twist my trunk as far to the right as possible and then all the way to the left, moving as rapidly as possible. Resistance is adjusted by moving forward or backward.
3. **Cable-machine crunches**
   3.1. I do straight-down crunches mixed in with side (oblique) crunches—three or four sets to fatigue.
4. **Hanging leg raises**
5. **Side lifts for obliques**
6. **Various types of sit-ups**
7. **Front and side planks**
8. **Daily stretching movements**

Chapter 19 - Strength Training with Body Movements

Body-weight movement is a major part of my strength training. In the list of my strength training movements in **Chapter 15**, I have listed body movements that I use. I summarize these below.

1. **Parallel dip.** This is a compound movement, but it mainly focuses on triceps and pecs.
2. **Push-up (many variations).** This is a compound movement, but it mainly works the triceps, pecs, lats, and core. I often use elastic bands for added resistance.
3. **Chin-up (various hand placements).** I often use elastic bands for resistance.
4. **Pull-up (various hand placements).** I often use elastic bands for resistance.
5. **Various sit-ups, crunches, leg raises, and planks.** I often use elastic bands for resistance.

6. **Heavy-bag boxing**. This requires multiple movements. I describe this exercise in detail in *Chapter 20*.

A new strength training approach appearing in various gyms is the TRX system. TRX refers to total-body resistance exercise, which uses gravity and your body weight for resistance movements. You anchor the portable TRX straps to a secure spot or a rack (now provided by most health clubs). I have not tried the TRX system.

PART 7

Combined Cardio and Strength Training

Effective Cardio Training during Strength Training Sessions

I would like to continue to separate my cardio and strength training sessions, as I believe this is the best way to obtain ***exceptional physical fitness***. However, my running cardio sessions are limited because of my knee problems, which are worsening as I age. So, I am interested in developing effective nonrunning cardio sessions (high average heart rate over a significant period) to go along with my strength training sessions. Some people say that the CrossFit approach effectively combines cardio training and strength training. But, as I noted earlier, I don't think that approach provides effective cardio workouts.

Below, I describe several approaches that I have examined in an effort to combine cardio training (without running) and my current strength training sessions.

Chapter 20 - Combined Cardio and Strength Training Sessions

When I tested whether any of the various types of strength training that I currently do (**Part 6**) would provide a significant cardio training, I found that ***none of my thirty- to forty-five-minute sessions of intense strength*** *training provided a significant average heart rate over the training period (using my Garmin heart rate monitor).* This is because the repetitions of a movement are not done in rapid succession. The rest time between each set and the time spent moving to the next equipment and setting up the weights allows significant heart rate recovery.

I have tried to introduce some type of *HIIT* to my strength training sessions by changing the resistance during sets and moving rapidly between sets and the next movement. This also did not work. Even at the maximum effort of a set, my heart rate was significantly below what I would see in a running or biking session.

Of course, using rapid reps and little rest time between sets is not an effective method of strength training. I do think the CrossFit training approach provides a cardio training effect, but that effect is much less than that of a separate cardio session as I pursue it.

CHAPTER 21 – PUSHUP CHALLENGE

SEVERAL YEARS AGO I HEARD a *Jack LaLanne* interview on a radio station as I was going to the gym. This was likely his last interview, as he was 96 years old at this time, but he came across very well! He died a year or so later. *Jack was one of my all time physical fitness heroes!* One of the many great things about *Jack* is that he is credited as being one of the first major physical fitness personalities to *introduce physical fitness training to women*! Also, *Jack* invented a lot of the current equipment in health clubs.

I was thirteen years old in 1957, living in Fort Sumner, New Mexico. We did not have a TV, so I would go down to the local hardware store, where, through the front windows, I would watch the big box TVs they were selling. It was there I first saw *Jack.* He was wearing black leotards, standing with two big dogs, and pushing a physical fitness class for women. Wow!

Jack realized that in order to be "fit," you needed to pursue a combination of cardio training and strength training. He was an exceptionally gifted swimmer, and swimming was his primary choice for cardio workouts.

Another one of my lifelong heroes is ***Arnold Schwarzenegger.*** Although he is considered the greatest bodybuilder of all time, he was not as physically fit as ***Jack***, as ***Arnold*** was totally focused on strength training. Going in the other direction, I don't consider world-class marathon runners or Tour de France winners, such as ***Lance Armstrong***, to be totally physically fit, either. But I do love ***Lance*** and ***Arnold!***

Jack did insanely crazy fitness stunts in the water from age forty to age seventy. He would handcuff his hands, shackle his legs, and tow five boats with seventy people aboard across several miles in the San Francisco harbor. The last time he did this, he was seventy.

Most of his fitness stunts were related to swimming and would be hard for somebody to repeat, especially if that person weren't a good swimmer, as I am not. However, ***Jack*** did perform several simple fitness movements that anyone could repeat.

In 1956, at age forty-two, ***Jack*** set a world record by doing 1,033 push-ups in twenty-three minutes (forty-five push-ups per minute) on ***You Asked for It,*** a television program hosted by ***Art Baker.*** So, I decided to see what I could do (even though I was thirty-one years older than Jack had been when he set his record). A second reason for my attempt, and more important, was that I wanted to determine what my average heart rate would be if I did push-ups for twenty to twenty-five minutes. ***The potential value here was that if my average heart rate was 70 percent to 80 percent of my maximum over the session, then I would have discovered another way - and a great way - to get an intense cardio workout without having to put pressure on my legs, knees, and the like.*** If I could achieve a high average heart rate from push-ups, which are strictly an upper-body movement (working the pecs, triceps, deltoids, traps, and lats and stressing the core), that would mean that I would not in any way be taxing my knees, which are rapidly wearing out.

I did not know how to pace myself, but I knew that *Jack* averaged forty-five push-ups a minute. *I can do seventy-five push-ups at one time (more if somebody is watching!),* but maxing out in the first minute or two is not the way to go. So, after doing thirty push-ups in the first thirty seconds, I settled on twenty to twenty-five push-ups with about a ten-second rest.

I was able to do 450 push-ups in twenty minutes (22.5 push-ups per minute). But, as noted, at this point, *I was thirty-one years older than Jack had been. Ha!*

My average heart rate (from my Garmin monitor) was a disappointing 112 beats per minute for the total workout of twenty minutes. But my maximum heart rate at the end of the twenty minutes was 131 beats per minute, which is about 85 percent of my maximum. What did I learn from this experiment? If I do a push-up "workout," I know I am not likely to get a high-level cardio workout. And doing push-ups for thirty or forty minutes would be hard to do and dull. The advantage to such a workout, however, would be that I wouldn't have knee pain. *This experiment was fun to do, and I plan to optimize it.*

CHAPTER 22 - HEAVY-BAG BOXING TRAINING

ONE OF THE MOST IMPORTANT physical fitness endeavors that I have used throughout my *sixty-seven years in pursuit of exceptional physical fitness* (and one that is still underway) is *"heavy-bag work"*. This refers to work with a punching bag. I believe heavy-bag punching is an excellent combination of cardio training and strength training. It embodies power movements—resistance plus speed.

On the farm, when I was six years old, Daddy set up a heavy bag for boxing training. Unfortunately, the bag was outside, and the weather affected the hitting surface.

At about ten years old, I decided to design my own bag. I got a green army duffel bag and filled it with a mixture of cottonseed and sawdust. This was great until it rained; when it got wet, the bag would harden, and hitting it was like hitting a tree. *For my workouts, I would get a baseball bat and practice my little league bating by hitting the bag, great! But, also softening up the bag for punching maneuvers.*

I have mixed heavy-bag workouts into my routine cardio and strength training programs ever since I left high school (in 1962). I always bought nice leather bags from Juarez, Mexico, about a hundred miles south of Roswell, New Mexico. I have continued to use heavy bags ever since, taking a bag with me everywhere I moved to. These were of high-quality leather, as were the boots I wore throughout high school and some years beyond. Hey, this is Roswell, where the aliens landed. *Ha! I don't believe any of that.*

Many years later, water-filled bags with polyethylene covering became the new and best technology. I have such a bag, and it can be filled with water to provide a total weight of about one hundred pounds. I fill my bag to an eighty-pound level and hang it from the rafters in the garage. I have worn out many of these bags over the years.

Eventually, I became engrossed in my BS and PhD studies, much the way I had pursued physical fitness in my early years. In my college days, I had to reduce my physical fitness efforts somewhat, but I did continue to carry and use my heavy bag, and *I still use it some sixty years later.* Back in those days, I also added a bench with a rack for a barbell. I carried these along with my heavy bag. At the colleges I attended - NMMI, ENMU (in Portales), the University of New Mexico (in Albuquerque), and finally Brigham Young

University (in Provo, Utah) - there were few, if any, established strength training gyms. Gold's Gym, 24 Hour Fitness, LA Fitness, and the like did not exist yet.

I became concerned with the mix of cardio and strength training. What was the best way to combine the two?

What would be the best cardio and strength training sessions, considering my age? This is discussed in **Parts 5 and 6.**

I had already determined that doing bag work or push-ups can get my heart rate up to a high level, but doing these movements for thirty minutes is tough and boring. But doing these exercises *after* getting my heart rate up to a high level from a running or biking session is a good way to go.

Heavy-bag training is relatively special in that it is an excellent combination of cardio and strength training. And, different from most strength training, it incorporates power movements, which involve a combination of resistance and speed, like throwing a baseball or football. Also, the strength training movements are highly compounded because multiple joints are necessary - legs, hips, shoulders, chest, back, biceps, triceps, and core. All punches are compound movements, but each type of punch has a major muscle movement. For example, the triceps are the major muscle used when throwing a left or right jab or a straight right or left punch, and these punches involve rapid core twists. Right and left hooks use the deltoids and biceps and, again, major core twists. Left and right uppercuts use shoulder and bicep movements.

Bag work can be compared to strength training with elastic materials, as it is a power movement. I currently use the bag just after a running or biking session. I go aggressively for two to three minutes with short rest periods, and then I do a set of push-ups, sit-ups, and pull-ups. I get a high average heart rate, about 80 percent to 85 percent of my maximum. I use right and left hand stances for best results.

Another great thing about bag work is that it is not a major stress on your knees, which is so important to me as I age. Another compound movement that combines cardio and strength training is rowing, but rowing does not work your core the way bag work does, and the knees are involved.

Unfortunately, 24 Hour Fitness clubs do not have heavy bags. When I asked them about this, they replied that they do not want to contribute violence. Ha! More likely, they do not want to deal with the expense of installing the bags. LA Fitness, Frogs, and most other fitness clubs have heavy bags but mainly for martial arts. ***If you are tough, these bags will work for boxing maneuvers.***

I must mention that one of the most valuable aspects of bag work is that it is functional training. This means that you are training at something that ***"can be of real value in real life, such as whacking somebody upside the head when they need it"***. I have certainly accomplished this!

PART 8

My Diet

You cannot possibly eat and drink all the items that the dietary literature suggests. Yet if you believe the scientific data about the value of raw fruits and vegetables and other nutritional items, taking fruit and vegetable extracts is supposedly a way to deal with this situation. I take extracts (described in **Part 9**) and certain fresh vegetables and fruits every day (discussed below).

I am not in any way against eating meat, but rarely do I have it in a meal. Maybe I do this because of the cost or the preparation. The most meat I get is buying a Subway sandwich with double meat every few months. One of these lasts me about five days. I do use chili beans with meat in my bean mix soup and chicken in my salad preparation. But I guess I'm pretty much a vegetarian.

How I Take In Fresh Fruits and Vegetables
Many food items have been determined to be nutritionally important. Considering this, I have decided to consume some of these foods in direct ways.

Into my spicy cheese dip, I dip a half a cup of fresh broccoli (steamed for three minutes to liberate the active ingredients) or a cup of spinach or high-fiber chips, like Beanitos. Broccoli and spinach are two of the highest-rated sources of antioxidants available. I do this every day.

I buy a big bag of frozen blueberries, put several cups in a bowl, and keep the bowl in the refrigerator. I have two tablespoons of these blueberries a couple of times a day. ***Blueberries are also one of the best available sources of antioxidants.*** Trying to consume fresh blueberries is expensive, and you end up with stale fruit, which is not appetizing.

I drink one or two cans of V8 juice a day. This is equal to several helpings of vegetables.

Most data indicate that the best way to consume vegetables and fruits is in their fresh and raw state. Some may be steamed, but getting your veggies from a can of vegetable soup is certainly not the best way to go.

BREAKFAST

Research suggests, and I believe, that the most important meal of the day is breakfast. I have a high-protein powder (30 g of CytoGainer, three cups of nonfat milk (27 g of protein), high-fiber raw tortillas (13 g of fiber and 8 g of protein), and one-third of a cup of salted and roasted edamame (13 g of fiber and 15 g of protein). The protein in this meal is about 80 g, about a half of the daily amount I would like to consume, considering my level of physical activity. Edamame are an outstanding food, offering complete protein, high amounts of fiber, and little fat. I order these from Amazon.

Overall, my daily intake of protein is about 140 g—about a gram per pound of body weight. This is a high level, but it meets my level of activity. I could take in more protein if I wanted to gain more muscle weight, but I'm happy with my current body weight.

FIBER

Considerable evidence supports the value of eating a diet rich in fiber, in particular as a key to aging successfully. According to a ten-year follow-up study, people who have the highest intake of fiber actually have an almost 80 percent greater likelihood of living a long and healthy life. That is, they are less likely to have hypertension, diabetes, dementia, depression, and functional disability. These findings suggest that increasing your intake of fiber-rich foods could be a successful strategy in remaining disease free and fully functional in your old age.

I particularly pay a lot of attention to getting fiber into my diet. The suggested amount is 25 g for women and 30 g for men. However, I don't think there is any way women or men can get these amounts from their usual diets. You have to work at this; read the labels, and pick foods that are high in fiber. The breakfast described above contains 25 g of fiber.

This issue was brought to my attention recently at my daughter's house. She had a package of buns, and each bun had 1 g of fiber. If she had selected the same brand of buns that were sitting on the shelf next to the first ones, she would have had a bun with 8 g of fiber. ***One of these buns would have provided about one-third of her daily requirement.***

Also, high-fiber foods are typically much better foods overall, with more protein, less fat, and so on.

I make sure my diet supplies about ***65 g of fiber and 140 g of protein a day.*** I don't think that there is any issue with having too much fiber. Likely, getting up to the suggested level of fiber intake will have some positive effect on your bowel movement, which I think is a good thing.

Whole Fruit versus Fruit Juice

It's tempting to think you can get one of your daily fruit servings from a glass of juice, but many researchers say you should skip the convenience and instead eat the whole fruit.

Years ago, I bought one of the ***Jack LaLanne Power Juicers***. However, I never took it out of the box. I had begun to realize that there was considerable value—fiber and the like - in the solid remains of the juice.

I should note that getting the nutritional value of fruits and vegetables by taking the extracts is much like taking the juices and not the fiber.

One study has found that eating more fruit—such as blueberries, grapes, and apples—is significantly associated with a lower risk of type 2 diabetes. Conversely, greater consumption of fruit *juices* is associated with a *higher* risk of type 2 diabetes.

NUTS

I have about half a cup of mixed nuts (walnuts, almonds, pistachios, peanuts, macadamia nuts, peanuts, and so on) each day. In addition, I also take in about one-fourth of a cup of walnuts a day. Walnuts have a special nutritional value, discussed below.

Nuts are a delicious part of an antiaging diet, helping ward off chronic diseases like cardiovascular disease, diabetes, and certain cancers.

After analyzing thirty years' worth of data, scientists linked eating one ounce (28 g, or approximately one-third of a cup) of nuts each day to a 20 percent reduced risk of death from any cause, including cancer, heart disease, and respiratory disease. There's strong evidence that eating nuts regularly can boost your health and your longevity.

Walnuts are particularly nutritional compared with other nuts. In addition to containing copper, folic acid, phosphorus, vitamin B$_6$, and manganese, walnuts contain high levels of a special form of vitamin E called gamma-tocopherol, which is most related to antioxidant effects. I specifically select the gamma-tocopherol tablets for my daily vitamin use. Walnuts are rich in omega-3 fats and contain greater amounts of antioxidants than most other foods. Eating walnuts may improve brain health while also helping prevent heart disease and cancer.

Further, because walnuts contain a complex mixture of bioactive plant compounds, they are exceptionally rich in antioxidants. In fact, walnuts ranked second in a study investigating the antioxidant content of 1,113 foods commonly eaten in the United States.

Nuts are easily incorporated into the diet, since they can be eaten by themselves or added to many different foods. ***Simply put, eating walnuts may be one of the easiest things you can do to improve your health.***

EDAMAME (GREEN SOYBEANS)

Soy protein is a high-quality, complete protein, which is key for performance in active and athletic people. It contains all the necessary amino acids for muscle building and repair. Many studies have shown that soy protein, much like the protein found in whey, can support increased muscle mass during resistance-type training. Soy protein is the only complete plant protein that is equivalent to animal protein.

Eating soy foods may help protect against prostate cancer. In fact, research suggests that regular consumption of soy foods may reduce the risk of prostate cancer by as much as 30 percent. A 2015 study analyzing isoflavone levels in the blood discovered that those individuals who consumed soy had the lowest likelihood of developing prostate cancer, and, even more, soy greatly reduced the risk of cancer metastasizing, or spreading throughout the body.

The roasted and salted edamame that I currently take with my breakfast and the raw shelled edamame I add to my soups both have 13 g of fiber and 13 g of complete protein per serving. Also, they have no cholesterol or trans fats.

In addition to raw edamame, I also use raw lima beans, lentils, and split peas in my soups and salads to provide additional fiber and protein.

I have been following the same diet for the past five years. ***Thus, it is time honored and value established, meaning that if in some way my diet were causing health problems, I would know about it.*** My weight has been constant at 143 (plus or minus a pound) over the past ten years, and my health has continued to be excellent. I do continue to modify my diet as I see important information from the literature. My current diet is outlined below.

BREAKFAST

1. One cup of black coffee
2. Two scoops of CytoGainer powdered protein (30 g). This has a significant amount of essential branched-chain amino acids, carbohydrates, vitamins, minerals, and creatine, so it's not just the usual protein powder.
3. I dissolve the powder in three cups of whole milk (30 g of protein).
4. One-third cup of edamame (15 g of protein)
    4.1. This contains 13 g of fiber.
        4.1.1. And it is a complete protein!
5. One tortilla (10 g of protein)
    5.1. This has 13 g of fiber.
        5.1.1. I use La Tortilla Factory Tortillas or Mission Flour Tortillas (Soft Taco).

Note that in my typical breakfast, I take in about 85 g of protein, which is a good amount for my level of physical activity, and about 27 g of fiber.

LUNCH, MIDDAY (ABOUT 10 G OF FIBER AND 35 G OF PROTEIN)

6. V8 juice (one or two cans)
7. One-third to one-half a cup of various types of nuts, particularly walnuts
8. Forty grams of whey protein and a creatine/amino acid formula
9. One pint of chocolate milk (22 g of protein)

10. One-third cup of raw blueberries
11. Various vegetables and fruits as described above

DINNER

12. I make a large salad, composed of about twenty ingredients, that lasts about two weeks.
    12.1. Some ingredients I use are spinach, lettuce, cabbage, celery, bell peppers, Bermuda onions, green onions, black olives, green olives, jalapeños, broccoli, carrots, radishes, tomatoes, hard-boiled eggs, raw soybeans, raw lima peas, walnuts, chicken, and blueberries.
       12.1.1. And I have one tortilla (13 g of fiber).
             12.1.1.1 Overall, I take in approximately 20 g of fiber at dinner.
    12.2. This "salad" is much more than just a salad, considering the protein and fiber content of the various ingredients.
13. I make a large container of soup that lasts about a week, composed of the following:
    13.1. Lentils, split peas, many types of beans, hominy, chili meat, and more.
       13.1.1. This provides about 10 g of fiber per serving and a considerable amount of protein.
14. I also have one cup of fresh spinach and one cup of fresh, steamed broccoli.
15. And I have two strong beers (***Steel Reserve 211, 8.1 percent alcohol***) and ***half a glass of cheap (boxed) wine.***
    15.1. I never have more, and often I have less.
16. I get about 5–10 g of fiber from general snack foods.
    16.1. This includes a serving of Beanitos with dip every day.
       16.1.1. One serving has 6 g of fiber—a great, healthy snack food.
17. ***Honey Pearl*** and Harley-Man (my "care dogs") and I share a small Drumstick ice cream every night.

So, in total, the fiber I take in every day is 60–70 g.

Again, this diet is time honored—over five years—so everything is going well.

Getting in a significant amount of fruits and vegetables every day is also hard to do.

You can't sit around all day and eat fruits and vegetables! Other than taking in raw blueberries, spinach, and broccoli, I take in fruit and vegetable extracts every day (discussed in **Part 9**).

I have followed this diet every day for the past five years with few changes.

PART 9

Supplements
Vitamins, Minerals, Herbal
Products, and Medications

ACCORDING TO RECENT RESEARCH, PEOPLE who use multivitamins and other nutritional supplements tend to lead healthier lives overall, so taking supplements can be seen as a positive.

I am a longtime, firm believer in taking various dietary supplements, such as vitamins, minerals, and herbal products. A long history of scientific research has demonstrated that antioxidants are useful in later life. I am a medicinal chemist and believe in long-established scientific research. I am betting that the research on antioxidants is correct, and I will continue to take supplements. Of course, you can find literature on many of the supplements that will not be too supportive, but the majority of the literature does strongly support taking supplements.

Everybody should devise his or her own supplement list by reading the literature. Of this list, a few will provide a notable effect within a few hours or within a few days. Others—such as vitamin C, vitamin D_3, vitamin E, calcium, magnesium, and omega-3 fatty acids - will not provide immediate detectable effects.

If I don't take my Aleve and Advil pills an hour before my running cardio session, I have considerable pain, to the point of getting a poor workout (low average heart rate). These pills offer a direct effect. Similarly, when I take my bronchodilator, albuterol, I quickly realize a positive effect on my breathing during cardio workouts.

You must have faith that many years down the road, you will derive healthful benefits from certain supplements.

Below, I provide a list of vitamins, minerals, and other supplements that I currently take or have taken over the years. I continue to change this list as new research is presented. After this information, I provide more details on select supplements.

1. **Vitamins and minerals**
   1.1. Vitamin C, 1,000 mg (one tablet) once a day
   1.2. Vitamin D_3, 5,000 IU (one tablet) once a day
   > *1.2.1.* It is highly likely that everybody reading this has a significant vitamin D_3 deficiency. Vitamin D_3 deficiencies are related to many medical problems. I mention more about vitamin D_3 below.

   1.3. Vitamin E, Vitamin E Factor Maxi-Gamma
   > *1.3.1.* Typical vitamin E supplements are in the alpha form, but the most important one is gamma-tropenol, which typically is not sold in stores. Order it online!

   1.4. Calcium, 600 mg plus 800 IU vitamin D_3 (one tablet) once a day
   1.5. Extend-release magnesium, one tablet per day
   1.6. LifeExtension High Potency Multivitamin & Mineral Supplement, two tablets per day

2. **Antioxidant extracts**
   2.1. Super Juice (vegetable, fruit, and botanical extracts), two tablets per day

2.2. Green tea extract, two tablets per day

2.3. Lycopene extract, one tablet per day

2.4. Blueberry extract, one tablet per day

    2.4.1. I also eat a quarter of a cup of fresh blueberries a day. I mention more about blueberries below.

2.5. JuiceFestiv fruit extracts

    2.5.1. These contain fruit extracts and other components.

        2.5.1.1 I have a capsule two times a day.

2.6. JuiceFestiv vegetable extracts

    2.6.1. These contain vegetable extracts plus five grains and greens.

        2.6.1.1 I take a capsule two times a day,

3. **Extracts for joints, mainly my knees**

    3.1. Triplex Flex (glucosamine, chondroitin, MSM)

    3.2. Glucosamine, chondroitin, MSM (liquid)

        3.2.1. I have taken supplements in an attempt reduce my arthritic knee pain. However, none have had any positive effect. Various scientific articles indicate that these materials typically are effective in only about 10 percent of the people taking these supplements. I am certainly in the 90 percent group.

    3.3. Advil (ibuprofen), 400 mg (two tablets) an hour before a cardio workout

    3.4. Aleve, 440 mg (two tablets) along with the Advil before cardio workouts

4. **Others**

    4.1. Fish oil, 1,000 mg (one capsule) two times a day

    4.2. Krill oil (MegaRed), one softgel tablet a day

    4.3. CoQ10 (Quinol—Active CoQ10), 200 mg per day

    4.4. Aspirin (Bayer Low Dose), 81 mg once a day

    4.5. Creatine/L-glutamine mixture: (1:1 powders, dissolved in water, kept in refrigerator), one-third of a cup of the supernatant liquid one to two hours before strength training

4.5.1. I mention more about this below.

4.6. Creatine X3, Elite Series, one scoop dissolved with water, one to two hours before strength training sessions

4.7. Whey Protein, Body Fortress, Super Advanced, one scoop (30 g of protein)

5. **Prescription drugs (to treat high blood pressure)**

   5.1. Zestril (lisinopril), 10 mg four times a day

      5.1.1. I have a family history of high blood pressure. I have taken this drug for about twenty years. It works, but what else is it doing? There are side effects related to its long-term use. Of these, I often have the "lisinopril cough," which occurs early in the morning.

6. **Other supplements**

   6.1. Years ago, Hydroxycut, a dietary supplement sold at various drug stores, was a great favorite of mine. I typically used it before my cardio workouts. Later, reports revealed that the formulation contained a significant amount of ephedra, a supplement banned by the FDA in 2004. It was soon taken off the shelves and later came back reformulated without ephedra.

   6.2. In my college days, you could go down to Juarez, Mexico, and freely buy methamphetamine, a derivative of ephedra. I did so several times. However, I never used it for any sort of enjoyment or physical fitness training, only for cramming for various tests.

   6.3. Supplements are available that claim to support the generation of human growth hormone (HGH). One that I have taken is Always Young. I do think this provides some good feeling during my day and helps in my workouts.

Vitamin D3

Vitamin D_3 is one of the most important natural vitamins and essential for many bodily functions. Insufficient concentrations are connected to many medical problems.

Research has shown that everybody has a vitamin D_3 deficiency. Unfortunately, you need to have a blood test to determine your actual level. Of course, as is typical in the area of supplements, there are reports that a vitamin D_3 deficiency is not a widespread problem.

After several blood tests, I found that even when I was taking a 5,000 IU tablet every day, my levels were barely over the suggested lower limit. Later, I realized that this vitamin, being fat soluble, should be taken with larger meals. Unfortunately, my meals typically do not contain a lot of fats. But I now take a 5,000 IU tablet of vitamin D_3 with a major meal. There is no evidence of toxic effects or overdosing from vitamin D_3.

I finally got my vitamin D_3 level to 99.5 ng/dl, the top of the prescribed range (of 30 to 100 ng/dl) for my age. No doubt this is because I take 5,000 IUs of vitamin D_3 a day *with my meals.*

A significant amount of vitamin D_3 can be obtained from the sun, but many variables affect the effectiveness of this method, such as temperature, length of exposure, amount of skin exposed, skin color, and so on. You should also consider the issue of skin cancer. I do get quite a bit of sun on my run and bike sessions, especially on my legs and arms, and I try to sit in the sun every day for twenty to twenty-five minutes. Apparently, this is not enough to get my vitamin D_3 level into the suggested range.

CREATINE

Much positive research over the past twenty years has demonstrated creatine's positive effect on strength training for muscle building, as well as on many other medical problems.

In 1993, about the time creatine was becoming known, I did an experiment to determine how many reps I could do with a specific weight movement (I chose the bench press). I then took creatine for two days before my next session. I found I could do ten reps, to fatigue, compared with eight reps in the previous session—a 25 percent increase! I have other strength training examples that clearly show that this supplement truly works.

Athletes use creatine to improve their overall performance, but creatine may also help treat a range of neuromuscular and neurodegenerative disorders, such as arthritis, Parkinson's disease, congestive heart failure, and depression, in addition to improving cognitive ability.

I have continued to use creatine over the years. I describe two ways I take it. The easiest is the ***Elite Series Creatine X3*** (available at Walmart), which has some other strength training components. I have just a scoop of the powder, in water, an hour before my strength training workout. As noted above, I also buy powdered creatine and glutamine and use a one-to-one mixture, dissolved in water at room temperature, and drink a third of a cup before my strength training sessions.

Creatine is the most common amino acid found in our muscles—over 61 percent of skeletal muscle is ***L-glutamine***. During intense training, glutamine levels are greatly depleted in the body, which decreases strength, stamina, and recovery. Studies have shown that glutamine supplementation can minimize breakdown of muscle and improve protein metabolism.

Creatine helps athletes with fast-twitch muscle fibers (used to swing a bat, run short dashes, or punch a heavy boxing bag) more so than athletes with slow-twitch muscles (used by long-distance runners). An endurance athlete does not typically use fast-twitch muscles; thus, creatine is not likely to be effective in such individuals.

PART 10
Record Keeping, Medical Issues, and Lab Work

CHAPTER 23 - RECORD KEEPING

I HAVE BEEN DILIGENTLY KEEPING accurate records of my workouts and physical fitness levels. This means that I have a great deal of data that can be effectively organized for analysis. In the past twenty years, I have found several excellent computer programs that allow me to collect, organize, analyze, and present my fitness data. These are discussed below.

THE ATHLETE'S DIARY
About twenty years ago, I started using the Athlete's Diary, a computer program in which you add your data in a fill-in format. The data is subsequently organized, analyzed, and graphed in various ways.

GARMIN CONNECT
My Garmin GPS watch/heart monitor, described in **Chapter 15**, does numerous things. I started using the computer application Garmin Connect for my Garmin Forerunner 405 CX in 2006. If I'm within fifteen feet of

my computer, my Garmin Connect wirelessly downloads all the data from a current workout to it. So, now I have electronic records of all my running and biking cardio fitness data, which I can view and analyze. The Garmin Forerunner 405 CX watch/heart monitor provides readouts of distance, time, distance versus time (pace), maximum and slowest speed, elevation gain, elevation, average heart rate, maximum heart rate, elevation levels graphed, temperature, wind speed and direction, percent humidity, outline of the course on a map, virtual training, and more.

I must note that of all the things my Forerunner monitors, as I carry out my cardio session, I want to see only (1) time thus far, (2) distance thus far, (3) instantaneous heart rate, and (4) average heart rate thus far. In the final readings, total time, total distance, average heart rate, and maximum heart rate are provided on the Garmin Connect program on my computer. The elevation gain for my running and biking sessions is provided, and I have found this information useful. A lot more information is downloaded to my Garmin Connect computer program and stored for my use, if necessary.

Upon viewing my Garmin Connect, I write down certain information in a notebook so that I am able to transfer select data to the Athlete's Diary and Word documents.

WORD DOCUMENT TABLE

I record my cardio and strength training data in a Word document table that I designed on my computer. The Athlete's Diary and Garmin Connect are primarily designed for cardio training data. The Word document table allows me to enter strength training data, too. This contains data from the Garmin Connect computer file that I transfer to the Athlete's Diary. I have displayed a page of this table from November 2016.

Word Document Table of Daily Workouts

Mon	Tues	Wed	Thur	Fri	Sat	Sun
31 RUN 2.76mi/17:05m/m 46:46min 116/130 47:00 8 Triceps 3 Core Movements	Nov 1 8 Shoulder 1 Core Movements	2 BIKE 8.2mi/11.8MPH 41:30min 468 EG 124/146 HeBa/PuUps/SiU 8:00 = 125/148 50:00 9 Leg Movements	3 RUN 2.83mi/16:42m/m 47:24min 111/118 47:00 8 Biceps 1 Core Movements	4 6 Push/Chest 1 Core Movements	5 RUN 2.6mi/17:20m/m 43:20min 105/113 43:00 6 Pull 1 Core Movements	6 7 Leg 1 Core Movements
7 BIKE 8.0mi/12.0MPH 40:00min 491 EG 128/153 HeBa/PuUps/SiU 8:00 = 126/160 48:00 8 Triceps Movements 3 Core Movements	8 6 Shoulder 1 Core Movements	9 RUN 2.6mi/17:12m/m 44:45min 114/128 45:00 8 Biceps 1 Core Movements	10 BIKE 8.6mi/11.8MPH 43:48min 473 EG 128/149 HeBa/PuUps/SiU 8:00 = 126/146 52:00 6 Push/Chest 1 Core Movements	11 8 Leg 1 Core Movements	12 RUN 3.2mi/17:46m/m 66:46min 106/1113 57:00 6 Pull 1 Core Movements	13
14 BIKE 8.0mi/12.0MPH 40:00min 411 EG 128/160 HeBa/PuUps/SiU 8:00 = 129/160 48:00 8 Triceps 3 Core Movements	15 8 Leg Movements	16 RUN 2.4mi/17:01m/m 40:48min 112/133 41:00 8 Shoulder 1 Core Movements	17 BIKE 8.0mi/11.8MPH 41:18min 539 EG 124/146 41:00 8 Biceps 1 Core Movements	18 8 Push/Chest Movements	19 RUN 2.6mi/16:02m/m 41:366min 114/135 HeBa/PuUps/SiU 8:00 = 124/148 50:00 8 Leg Movements	20 6 Pull 1 Core Movements
21 RUN 2.6mi/16:66m/m 44:12min 116/133 44:00 2 Triceps 1 Core Movements	22 Blood Pressure Walmart 121/74/74	23 BIKE 9.59mi/11.9 MPH 48:15min 706 EG 126/147 56:00 8 Leg 1 Core Movements	24 6 Biceps Movement	25 RUN 2.6mi/17:30m/m 46:26min 110/123 46:00 8 Shoulder 1 Core Movements	26 8 Push/Chest 1 Core Movements	27 8 Leg 1 Core Movements

The various strength training movements are described in **Part 6**. In the table, RUN and BIKE denote my running and biking cardio sessions. I typically list the distance covered, minutes per mile for running, miles per hour for biking, average heart rate, maximum heart rate, percent incline gained, and total time for the running or biking session. **HeBa/PuUps/SiU** denotes heavy-bag work, push-ups, pull-ups, sit-ups, and the average heart rate and maximum heart rate of these parts. The total time on the complete cardio session is also listed.

Upon examining these documents, I can evaluate how my physical fitness levels have changed over the past twenty years.

For example, I can determine that the average time for my running sessions has increased from eleven minutes per mile to over fifteen minutes per mile, and biking sessions have decreased from sixteen miles per hour to about ten miles per hour. I should note that the high running times are due to my ***HIIT*** approach, which is a combination of less intense (fast walking) effort and more intense (slow jogging) effort. The overall pace of a ***HIIT*** session is not the important issue—***the average heart rate for the session is.***

Also, the courses I ran and biked twenty years ago are flatter than the hilly courses I am now using in the Cardiff, California, area, so a direct comparison is hard. Currently, I select biking courses with hills. As noted, the hills are about 250 to 300 yards long and are the intense portion of my ***HIIT*** workouts. And recently, I have introduced a final sprint in my running and biking sessions, which does increase my heart rate.

My average heart rate for cardio sessions has decreased from about 130 to about 120 beats per minute. But my maximum heart rate has also decreased, from 165 to 155. So, I am still getting about 80 percent of my maximum heart rate in my cardio training sessions. My weight has decreased from about 150 to 143 pounds. The Athlete's Diary shows how the objective of my workouts has changed; instead of participating in social or competitive events, I am now more concerned with physical fitness goals. My weight lifting maximums have come down somewhat. My body-weight movements, such as push-ups, pull-ups, dips, and sit-ups, have remained about the same.

CHAPTER 24 - MEDICAL ISSUES AND INJURIES

I HAVE BEEN RELATIVELY FREE of any serious medical problems. However, I do have some typical problems, described below.

Benign Prostatic Hyperplasia (BPH)

This section is for the guys. The prostate-specific antigen (PSA) test is a blood test commonly used to help predict prostate cancer. PSA is a protein that is made only by the prostate gland, and an increase beyond normal levels is a possible indication of the presence of prostate cancer.

Below, I describe a surefire way to reduce your BPH level.

First, here are some important facts. About 50 percent of men who are fifty years old are experiencing prostate problems, mainly voiding problems (*voiding* is the appropriate medical term for peeing or urinating), and 60 percent of men who are sixty years old are experiencing problems. And so on.

In 2011, my PSA level was tested at 7.5—well outside the normal range (0.0–4.0) and strongly suggestive of prostate cancer (according to many doctors). However, I had ridden thirty miles (about two hours) on my bike the day before the test, and this, like having sex the night before the test, should not have been done. Since there were no other negative problems, such as voiding problems, no action was taken.

In 2012, my PSA level was 5.5, and my urologist decided I should be assayed for possible prostate cancer. This was done by taking samples of my prostate from various sites by positioning a tube up my urethra, with additional monitoring by an instrument inserted in my rectum. Ho, fun! But I experienced no pain, as I was out, under painkillers. This was my first time in a hospital, and it lasted only four hours. I suppose that's pretty good for my age. All the tests for cancer were negative, but obviously I did have BPH.

Then, in early 2013, I began to experience voiding problems. I was not able to empty my bladder completely, and thus I had to void frequently—such as every hour and a half to two hours at night.

My urologist decided to check my prostate again. He found it to be enlarged; it was larger than a walnut when it should have been about the size of a grape. He decided to perform a transurethral resection (TURP). Guided by instruments through my rectum, the surgeons went through my urethra and used radiation to destroy and remove about half of the prostate. I was negative for prostate cancer.

This surgery helped a lot; still, on average, I had to void about every two hours. Sometimes, I would get three or four hours of sleep. Maybe my ability to ignore the urge related to how tired I was. The urologists told me that it could take a year to obtain the best result.

At the end of 2013, I got my blood tests back. My PSA value was 1.5. That was a significant drop from the past two years of 7.5 and 5.5. However, my voiding problems were still present. Thus, I had another TURP in 2015 to reduce a significant portion of my prostate. This has certainly helped, but I still have problems with voiding. The samples taken from my prostate were again negative for cancer. I hope things will get better as I age.

KNEE PROBLEMS

I have pain in my knees, which has gradually increased over the past twenty years. I think the pain is due to my body type (short and stocky), arthritis, and the old football injury. My father had both knees replaced at the same time in Juarez, Mexico, when he was in his seventies. He was a tough old guy who worked hard on the farm. My sister has had both knees replaced. She has been overweight most of her life, so the surgery made sense for her. When my mother was ninety-seven, she broke her hip getting into her car to go to her hairdresser, but she survived. *That is unbelievable for someone her age, or even for a sixty-five-year-old!* She is *now one hundred and mentally alert*, and she gets around with a walker. My father broke his hip at ninety and died in the hospital several days later. So, maybe I have some good genes. *But I am not counting on this. I will continue my pursuit of exceptional physical fitness.*

As noted earlier, I take 400 mg of Advil Liqui-Gels (ibuprofen capsules) about one hour before my cardio workouts. Recently, I have added two Aleve tablets (220 mg each). I am looking for any medical evidence that supports—or does not support—combining these over-the-counter painkillers. Currently, I do four or five cardio sessions a week. These are the running and biking workouts I described in part 5. These are intense—about forty-five to sixty minutes at about 80 percent of my maximum heart rate. Biking is great; I have no pain whatsoever. But running is difficult and causes a lot of pain. However, by doing high-intensity interval training (walking fast, jogging slowly, and repeating) and speed play, I can get a good training effect in. I don't know how long this will last, but I think I can bike forever, as I do not experience any pain.

Biking provides a huge mechanical advantage because most of your weight is on the bike seat. In running, your whole body hits the ground with every step—on one leg! Biking is great, but I have to push much harder to get a training effect.

My cardio sessions start with a mental test. I ask myself, *"Can I do this?"*

I typically don't take additional Advil and Aleve during the day. I do have pain during the day, but I just gut it out. Obviously, I will not be able to do this forever. I do wear black elastic knee bands for my runs. I probably should wear these sometimes during the day.

I have taken a ton of glucosamine, chondroitin, and MSM in numerous ways over the years, as noted earlier. However, I have never received any noticeable relief or help. Studies have shown that only about 10 percent of the people taking these supplements have any relief. For sure, I must not be in this 10 percent.

ASTHMA

I was first diagnosed with asthma in *1957*, when I was in the seventh grade. I would experience breathing problems, shortness of breath, coughing, wheezing, and chest tightness when I was around dust, grass, and other irritants. I took desensitization shots once a week for several years and then reduced the frequency to every two weeks. With the shots, I was quite normal, but if I missed a session, I had difficulty breathing. I took the shots throughout high school and then quit in my early college years, as my allergies seemed to go away. I was told that they might come back in later years. This was certainly the case—I began to have asthma symptoms in the early *1990s*. So, again, under the guidance of an allergy specialist, I began to take albuterol, a bronchodilator inhalant, which works by relaxing and opening the air passages to the lungs.

This worked well as long as I took the drug as prescribed. But in 2010, I quit taking the drug on a regular basis (as prescribed). Instead, I would take three inhales thirty to forty-five minutes before a running or biking cardio session. This certainly had a positive effect on my average heart rates. I noticed several years ago in the prerace literature for a popular triathlon in Oceanside, California, that albuterol was considered a performance-enhancing drug and was not allowed in the race. Yet I still saw several aerosol inhalants being passed from one competitor to another at the start of the run. I continued taking albuterol before my cardio session for several more years because of the positive effect on my average heart rate, but I have stopped taking it in the past three or four years.

CHAPTER 25 - LAB WORK AND BODY WEIGHT

IN MY JUNIOR COLLEGE DAYS, when I pumped up to 165 pounds for football and down to 140 for boxing, my body weight was around 150 pounds for years. But in the past ten years, it has been 143, plus or minus a pound. I always weigh myself at the same time—after each of my cardio sessions—and it never changes. This is expected, as my diet and workout program rarely change. However, recently, I've noticed a slight increase; my weight is now a constant 144 to 145 pounds.

What caused this increase? Because I wanted to make sure that any fat-soluble vitamins (such as A, D_3, E, and K) and my blood pressure medication, lisinopril, were being absorbed appropriately, I increased my fat intake. I determined that the food that could provide a reasonable increase in fat in my diet was milk, as I drink it every morning with my CytoGainer protein powder for breakfast. For years, I used fat-free milk, but for the past several months, I have been using whole milk, which contains 9 g of fat per serving (one cup). I take in three cups each morning, which is 27 g of fat. I believe this fat increase is responsible for my two-pound weight gain. What if I had a cheeseburger with fries every evening?

I have had my body fat percentage taken numerous times, with water-emersion and skinfold-calipers tests. It has always been lower than 10 percent.

BLOOD PRESSURE

My blood pressure has been above normal for most of my adult life. This is surprising, considering my lifestyle. However, my parents and most of my other family members have also had abnormal blood pressure, so this is likely a hereditary condition. I have taken blood pressure medication for the past twenty-five years. Currently, I take lisinopril, 40 mg a day. Lisinopril is an angiotensin-converting enzyme (ACE) inhibitor used primarily in the treatment of high blood pressure or heart failure and after heart attacks. It keeps my blood pressure at acceptable levels. In the past several years, my average blood pressure has been about 115/66, and my resting pulse has been fifty to fifty-five beats per minute. This is well in line with the recently revised optimal levels of blood pressures. I researched and bought a high-end blood pressure measurement apparatus several years ago so that I can reliably record my blood pressure at home. I also check my blood pressure at the machines at Walmart and Vons. The readings are usually close to the results I get at home. However, my blood pressure readings taken at the doctor's office are always high. Could this be the white coat effect?

MEDICAL TESTS

Every several years, I have a variety of lab tests taken by Life Extension. All values have been within the suggested levels, except my vitamin D_3 levels. As noted above, I have just recently managed to get my level near the maximum limit.

PART 11

Mental Aspects of Physical Fitness Training and My Physical Fitness Heroes

Chapter 26 - Mental Aspects of Physical Fitness Training

I THINK THERE ARE TWO types of people concerning physical fitness. First are the ones who enjoy working out and look forward to their workouts. ***This is me!*** I enjoy my physical fitness endeavors; of course, I have been doing this since I was six years old. My father was a committed athlete in football, boxing, and other sports, and we connected strongly in these areas. The other type people are the ones who don't enjoy physical fitness workouts. But many of them realize that they need to do *something*. So, there is a constant battle within these people; they try to force themselves to do what they know is best for them, but they don't want to do it. I don't know how everyone fits into these two types, but I suspect that most people do not enjoy workouts. However, if you are diabetic or significantly overweight, have high cholesterol levels, lack energy, and so on, a physical fitness program may be the best thing you can do. ***Actually, it may be essential.***

A recent study found that variation in genes for dopamine receptors, as well as in some other neural-signaling genes, helps explain why about 25 percent of participants drop out of exercise programs or don't exercise at the recommended level. The study suggested that these genes, combined with personality factors, might help explain why some people have a natural urge to be active while others never do.

I firmly believe *that I have maintained my lifelong pursuit of exceptional physical fitness mainly for my enjoyment, not to enhance my longevity or my physical well-being and appearance.*

We all have a book inside us, but we have to get it out and write it. From my experience in writing this book, it is a serious mental endeavor—at least, it was for me. *I have had to say continually, "OK, let's do this" and push myself to do it.*

I don't know why I have been able to carry out my physical fitness efforts over the years. Even after I've looked into many scientific studies that have focused on trying to identify and understand factors that lead to appropriate physical fitness, I have no answers.

Religion? - I am not at all a religious person. I certain believe in God, but do not go to church and I am not in any way active in church functions. On the other hand, the Cook family is very strong, active Southern Baptists. However, every day that I return from a cardio high intensity internal training (**HIIT**) sessions, *I do thank God for giving me the mental will power to complete such an intense workout!* And, I dearly hope that I can continue/maintain my *exceptional physical fitness* activities.

I do believe that it is a person's mentality that drives his or her physical fitness.

It is clear that my mind is related to my physical fitness endeavors in my cardio sessions of running and biking. Running is more strenuous than biking. In biking, most of your body weight is supported on the bicycle seat. Because of this mechanical advantage, it is much easier and quicker to derive a significant cardio event (high average heart rate for a reasonable period) from running than it is from biking. To acquire a comparable cardio event from biking, you must push harder. You can ride for fifteen or twenty miles and say, ***"Wow, I got a good workout in!"*** But when you look at your heart rate monitor, you'll see that your average heart rate over the ride was significantly less than it would be in a typical running session. This is not good. At my level of physical fitness, I would consider such a ride a waste of time.

The best way I have found to make biking as intense as running is knowing what my target average heart rate is for a running session and trying to match this in my biking session. Of course, the only reliable way to accomplish this is to use a heart rate monitor. When you know what values you need to achieve to match a running session, doing so becomes a mental feat. One of my approaches to this difference in cardio sessions is to bike up hills, which requires significant energy output. Failing and having to stop and turn your bike around is typically not a safe way to go, so getting to the top is your only option. In running up the hill, you can just walk slowly to get to the top, if you choose.

When I run hills, my heart rate goes up, and I have less knee pain. Unfortunately, I have to come down, and that's when my heart rate goes down and my knee pain goes up. I try to select running courses that have reasonable uphills and downhills to compromise on my heart rate and knee pain.

Considering my cardio sessions, I am a committed early morning person. I have a cup of coffee and a bit of a high-fiber protein bar or a cup of mocha cappuccino milk, which is an excellent before- and after-workout drink. Then, I hit the road between seven and eight. Rarely do I initiate a cardio session much later than eight. After a morning session, ***I typically feel that I have already accomplished something important and have a positive attitude throughout the rest of the day.***

I have found that ***the best time for me to think clearly is while biking or running, when there are no distractions.***

Sometimes, rarely, early in my run, I'll decide that I don't feel like running. Then, my knees begin to pain me a little, to support my mental decision. Ha! This is just another mental aspect of my physical fitness training.

It is quite rare that I ever skip a scheduled workout session. As noted in parts 5 and 6, my cardio and strength training sessions are well laid out. If I do miss a scheduled workout, I typically am bothered during the day and tend to increase my efforts in the next scheduled workout.

Also, on rare occasions, I feel that I will not get a good effort in if I follow my scheduled workout. Whenever I do a workout at a reduced level, I feel it is mainly a waste of effort and time and that I am just torturing myself.

Bear Bryant of the University of Alabama said, ***"It is not the will to win that matters. Everyone has that. It's the will to prepare to win that matters."*** The mental aspect of physical fitness is the overriding elephant in the room.

I just watched the 2016 NBA finals between the Cleveland Cavaliers and the Golden State Warriors. Well, the Cavs won—not my team, unfortunately. In the seventh game of the seven-game series, ***the Splash Brothers—Klay Thompson and Stephen Curry***—did not perform well, compared with their usual seasonal games. They missed too many three-point shots that they had made throughout the season and in previous games in the series. Why? If they had been seriously guarded, then it would've made sense, but they were not. Was this is a mental situation? Yes!

In another mental situation, in a recent game, ***Stephen Curry*** set an NBA record by knocking down thirteen three-pointers in a win over the New Orleans Pelicans. His shooting spree came one game after the two-time MVP missed ten shots from three-point range in a loss to the Los Angeles Lakers.

Another interesting aspect of my mental capabilities is that although I am an intense physical fitness devotee, ***I must note that it was hard for me to have reasonable periods of concentration when pursuing the writing of this book.***

I will guarantee that I will not be overweight when I am done here on this earth. I have often said to my family that if there are any burial procedures, I want to be observed in a Speedo. But I have a long way to go.

CHAPTER 27 - MY PHYSICAL FITNESS HEROES

I CONSIDER A HANDFUL OF sports people to be my heroes, and they have surely had some effect on my pursuit of exceptional physical fitness. I note these below, starting with my early years.

As noted, I often sat with my father on the farm to listen to *The Wednesday Night Fights* on the radio. This was one of the first national radio sports broadcasts. I didn't identify with any of the fighters, but my father did.

BOXING

I loved boxing, particularly when I could watch all the important fights on TV. But, hands down, I always followed the heavyweight division. I liked **Mike Tyson's** enviable destruction of his opponents. Yet my all-time favorite was **Muhammad Ali (Cassius Clay).** I tried to watch all his fights. Even when I was living in Ann Arbor, Michigan, I drove to Detroit and watched televised fights at several large event centers. Ali was known for various quotes. One I have enjoyed is, *"Float like a butterfly, sting like a bee."* Unfortunately, as I was writing this book, he passed away at the age of seventy-four. There was a huge outpouring of support for him. I must also note my great love for **Howard Cosell.** Of course, Cosell was not a fighter, **but he was a great ring announcer who spent a lot of time with Ali** and always generated much discussion.

BASKETBALL

Somehow, back in the early days, my favorite professional basketball team was the Boston Celtics. My favorite players then were **Bob Cousy, John (Hondo) Havlicek, and Bill Russell** - all members of the Celtics. They were the dominant team. I even tried to name my firstborn boy Havlicek, but my wife wouldn't go for it. But in 1968, I did name our first dog **Russell**. Much later, I was a big fan of the Detroit Pistons, as they won several titles during the time we lived in Ann Arbor,

Michigan, where I worked for Warner-Lambert/Parke-Davis. My favorite player in the league was the Pistons' ***Isiah (Zeke) Thomas.*** I was also a big fan of *Jerry West,* the Logo, who spent his whole career with the Los Angeles Lakers as a player and executive and was responsible for bringing **Kobe Bryant and Shaquille O'Neal to the Lakers.** Also in that period, I had season tickets to the University of Michigan Wolverines and got to see the **Fab Five** perform. I enjoyed **Bobby Knight**, from Indiana University. Some of his famous quotes are below:

> *"You don't play against opponents; you play against the game of basketball."*

> *"When my time on earth is gone, and my activities here are passed, I want them to bury me upside down, and my critics can kiss my ass!"*

For the past fifteen years, I have been a serious **Kobe Bryant** fan and, of course, a fan of the Los Angeles Lakers. I loved **Chick Hearn**, the announcer for the Lakers for so many years. I will certainly continue to support the team even though Kobe has retired, but I also like the Golden State Warriors, particularly the **Splash Brothers**. Just recently, **Kevin Durant**, being a free agent, signed with the Warriors. **Steve Kerr** has a big job in getting the best from all these all-stars. I do admire **Phil Jackson**—pro player, coach, general manager, author, and more—and still follow him even though he left the Lakers to go back to his original team, the New York Knicks.

FOOTBALL

My early football hero was *Johnny Unitas* of the Baltimore Colts, and I certainly followed **Roger Staubach** of the Dallas Cowboys. As I mentioned earlier, Roger was two years ahead of me at the New Mexico Military Institute. Today, I follow the San Diego Chargers (now the Los Angeles Chargers), especially **Philip Rivers**. Also, I must say that I did like **O. J. Simpson.**

GOLF

Early on, I followed *Arnold Palmer* and *Lee Trevino*; later, I followed *Tiger Woods*. I do not follow any specific player now, and *I must say that I have never played a round of golf in my life. I'm not old enough yet!*

TENNIS

John McEnroe and *Jimmy Connors*—I loved those guys! I watched all their matches, particularly when they played each other. I'm not following anybody now.

BASEBALL

I'm not a big baseball fan, but *Yogi Berra* of the Yankees was my favorite. Not only was he a great player, but he also came out with many interesting quotes, such as, *"When you come to a fork in the road, take it."* I also followed the Los Angeles Dodgers for a lot of years. And I loved *Vin Scully*, the announcer, who just retired. I also followed *Pete Rose* and his manager, *Sparky Anderson*, of the Cincinnati Reds.

BIKING

I'm happy to note that I'm a great supporter of *Lance Armstrong*. I view him as one of the greatest endurance athletes of all time. Yes, he took drugs, but everybody else in professional biking did as well during the days he competed. If you did not take drugs, you would not even be in the race. *If Lance and all the other pro cyclists had not taken any drugs, Lance would still have won.* His main problem was that he was so insistent on trying to hide the illegal drug use. To this day, I still wear two yellow *Livestrong wristbands (it's been thirteen years since 2004) - one because he is the greatest endurance athlete of all time, and one for his huge contributions to cancer research.*

BODYBUILDING

I just love *Arnold Schwarzenegger*. He has accomplished so much, and he is still going. He is an Austrian American actor, filmmaker, businessman, investor, author, philanthropist, and activist, as well as a former professional bodybuilder and former politician. He has been successful in most of these areas. He was surely not a great governor of California, but for sure he is the greatest bodybuilder of all time. Donald Trump made Arnold the emcee of *The New Celebrity Apprentice*!

JACK LALANNE

Jack will be missed by many, certainly by me, but his legacy will live on. Some of his quotes that I will always remember include the following:

"The only way to hurt the body is not use it."

"Your waistline is your lifeline."

"Ten seconds on the lips and a lifetime on the hips."

When he was ninety-four, *Jack* was asked on a radio program if he thought he'd live to be one hundred. His answer was to the point:

I don't care how old I live! I just want to be living while I am living! I have friends who are in their eighties, and now they're in wheelchairs or they're getting Alzheimer's. Who wants that? I want to be able to do things. I want to look good. I don't want to be a drudge on my wife and kids. And I want to get my message out to people.

He smiled before continuing. *"I tell people, I can't afford to die. It would wreck my image."*

DECATHLONS

I don't have any particular name here, but I do love decathlons. I think this event is an excellent example of the effective combination of cardio and strength training efforts.

Looking Forward

What Do I Expect Going Forward?

I am happy with my overall cardio and strength training sessions and my current level of physical fitness, *which I believe is exceptional.*

My cardio training sessions are as aggressive as I can provide, and I continue to try to increase their intensity. I carefully monitor my training sessions with my Garmin heart monitor. I often worry that my current monitor will eventually wear out or break, and so I have bought a backup. However, my current monitor has long been out of production, and many new models are available. My current Garmin does about twenty-five things, but I use only about eight. The new heart rate monitors probably do fifty things and can be connected to an iPhone, which I don't use. The Athlete's Diary and Garmin Connect are excellent computer-based methods to collect my data and analyze it. I certainly will continue with these systems.

I know my knees will eventually give out. I expect this will gradually happen in the next five years, probably sooner. I don't think that I will be interested in knee replacements. What will I do to replace my basic cardio sessions of running? Well, I think I can bike forever! If I lose some balance on the bike, I can use stationary bikes and go to spin classes. After that, I could resort to swimming. Yuck! I think my paddles for jogging in water, discussed in *Chapter 8*, would be a great way to get in significant cardio workouts. However, I certainly am not looking forward to this.

I am happy with my current strength training program and will continue to follow it. I do plan to add more work with elastic materials as time passes. Also, I plan to develop more sessions that combine cardio and strength training and still maintain high average heart rates.

I have utilized few stretching or balance sessions thus far in my workouts. I plan to gradually introduce various aspects of these as I get older.

I also have some interest in entering some biking events at my old age.

I think I have developed an excellent diet, one that is nutritional and affordable and that will change as I learn more. Maybe I should drink less beer, or maybe I should drink more beer. I'm joking; my alcohol intake is not a problem. In fact, much of the current literature supports my level of alcoholic intake.

My supplement use will certainly continue, and it will change, likely monthly, as I learn more from the literature.

I truly don't see a need to change my current physical fitness program, but I will keep alert to the developing literature.

> ***Whereas I say to others, "It is never too late," I say to myself, "Just keep it up!"***

So far, for sixty-seven years, for some reason (God's guidance, good genes - *something*), I have been able to effectively pursue a physical fitness program that has allowed me ***to be exceptionally physical fit throughout my whole life…and counting!***

> ***Like Jack LaLanne, I want to be living while I am living.***

Thus, I do plan to continue appropriate physical fitness endeavors, as much as possible, and to be ***exceptionally physically fit until the end.***

PART 13

What I Look Like at
Age Seventy-Three

I HAVE PROVIDED CURRENT PICTURES of me at age seventy-three. This is surely appropriate considering that you have spent several hours reading about *my pursuit of exceptional physical fitness*. It makes sense that you would want to see the so-called final product. These are not *Arnold Schwarzenegger* bodybuilding poses, just reasonably relaxed pictures.

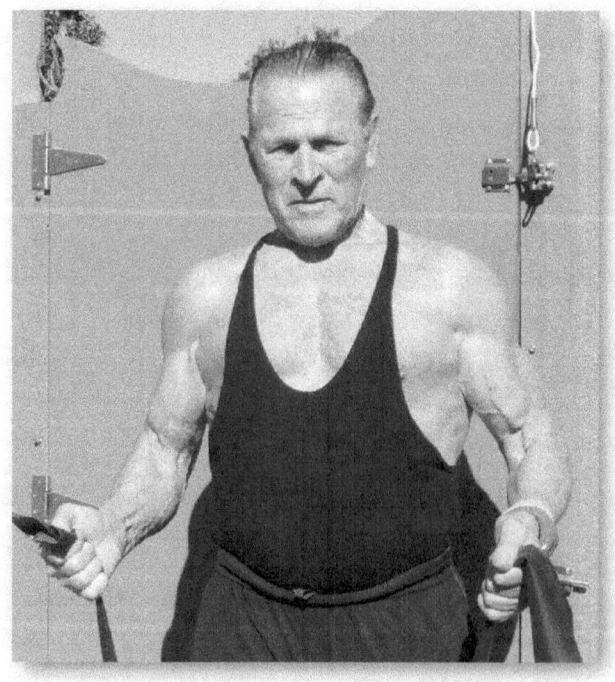

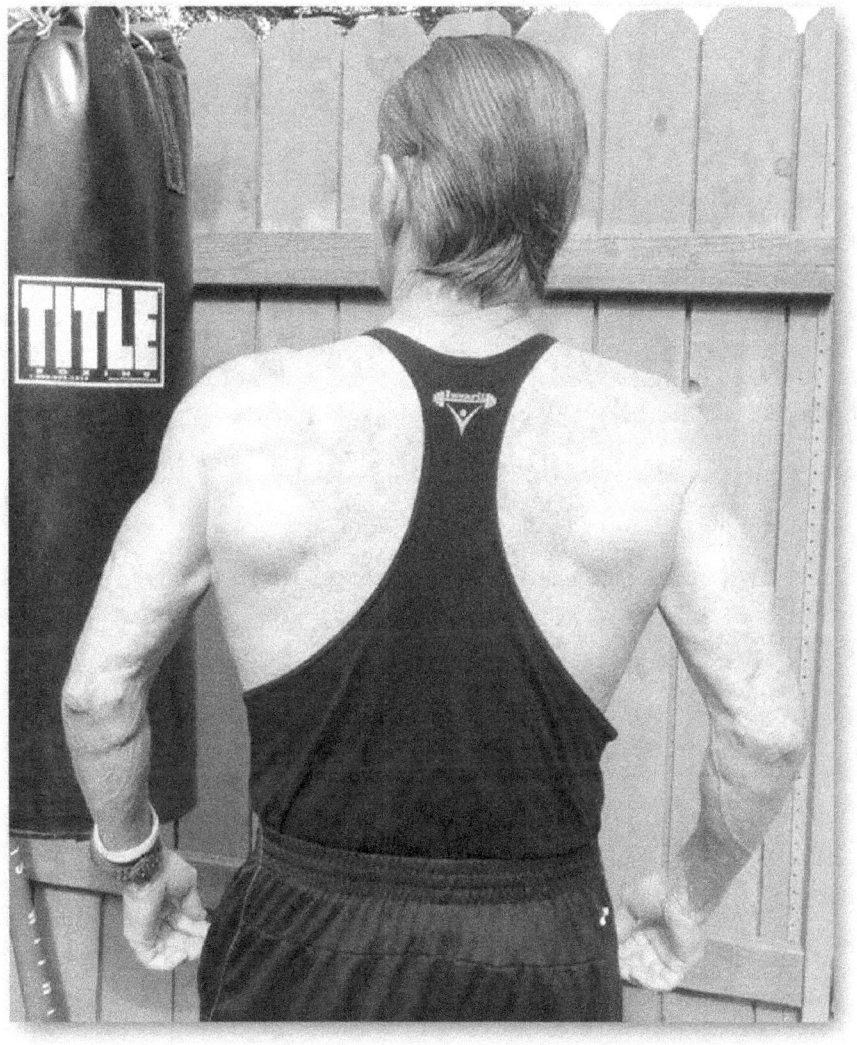

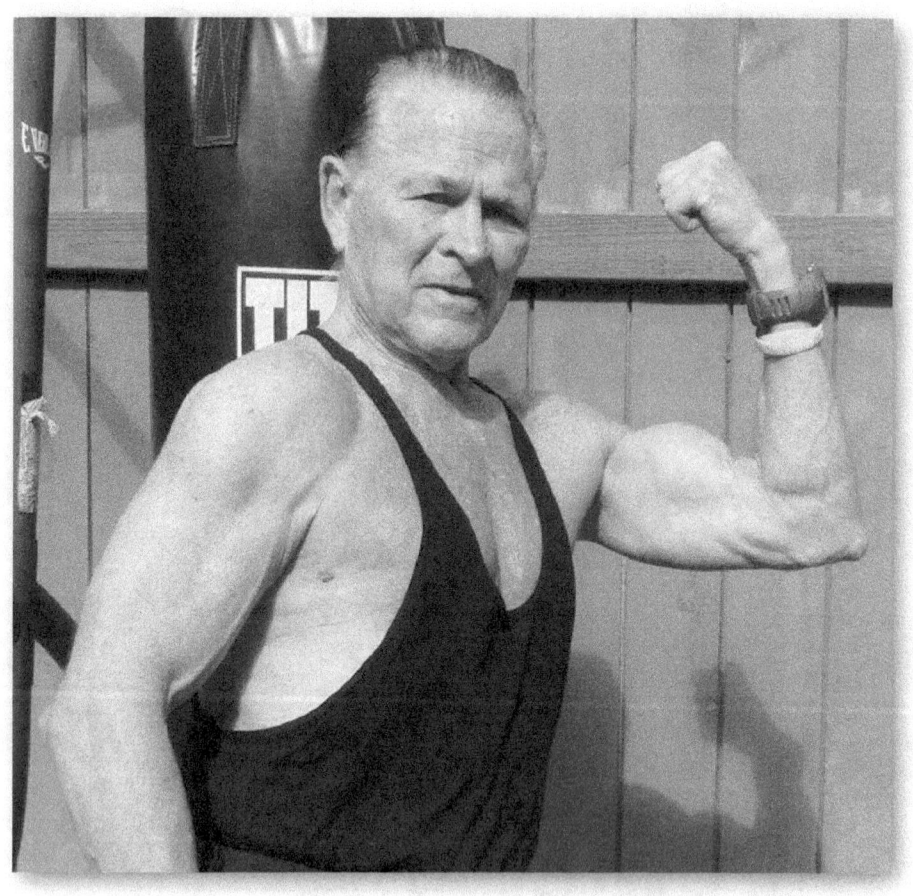

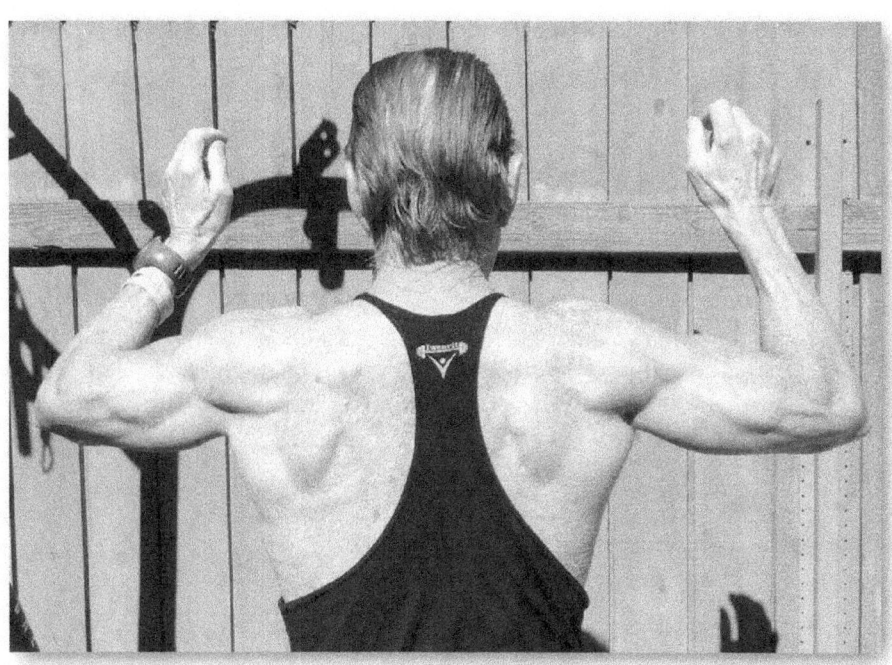

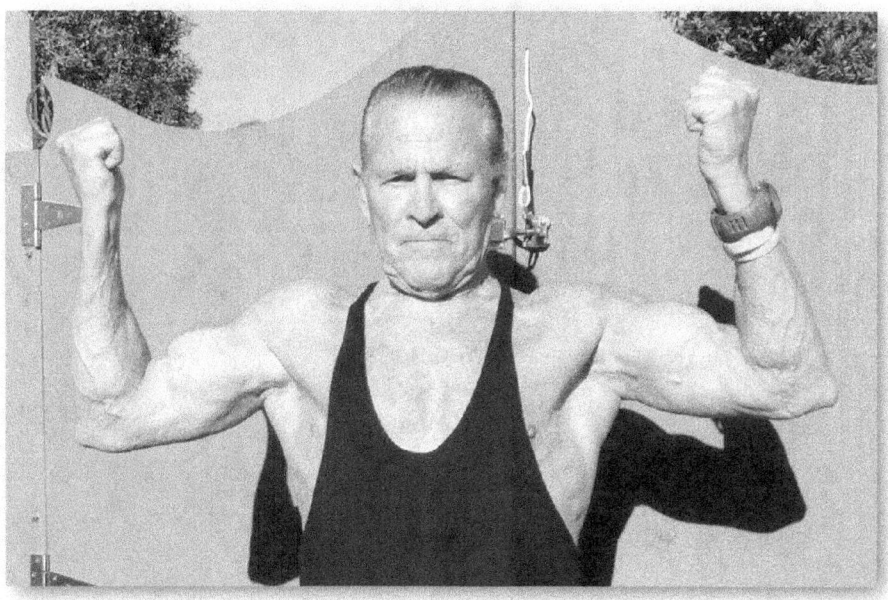

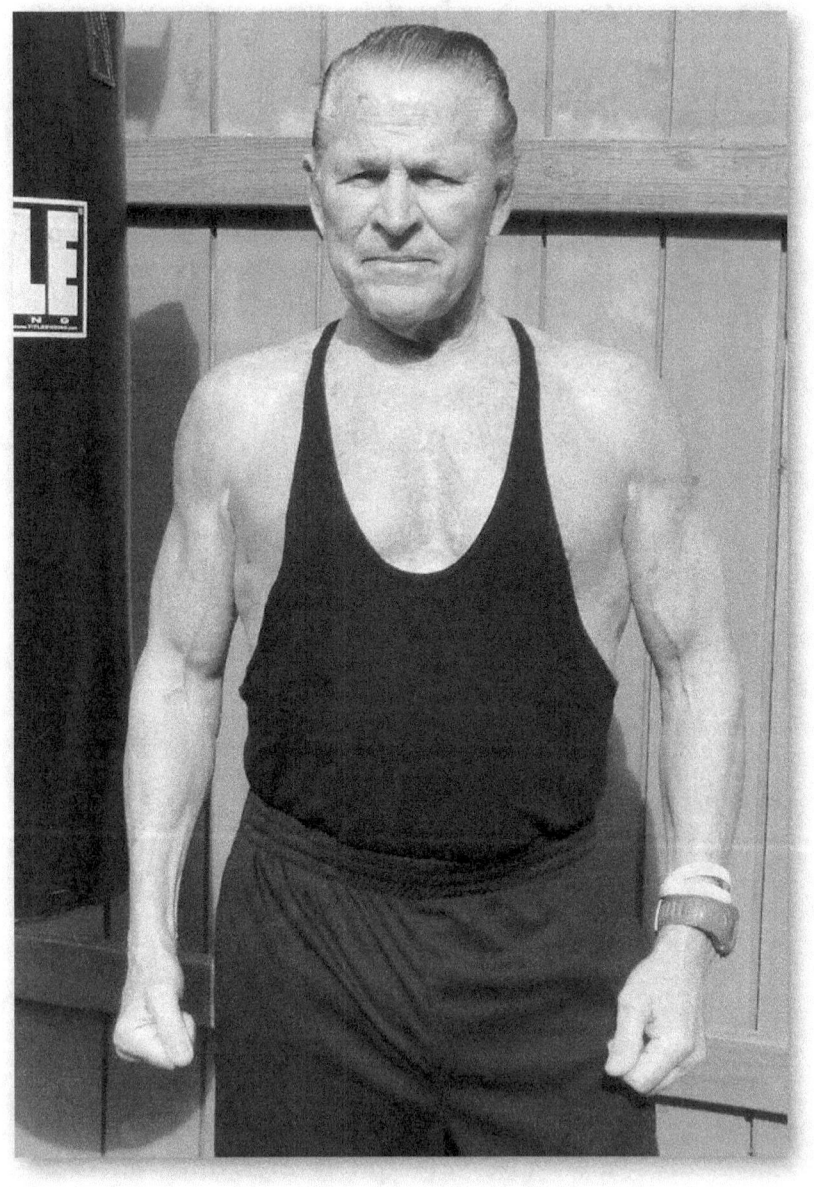

AUTHOR BIOGRAPHY

PHILLIP DAN COOK, PhD, ACE, NASM, has been a fitness enthusiast and advocate for his whole life. Now in his midseventies and retired, he continues to engage in running, biking, resistance training, and boxing workouts despite hypertension, arthritic knees, prostate problems, and exercise-induced asthma.

Cook holds a doctorate in medicinal chemistry. Prior to his retirement, he served as a drug-discovery executive, senior research director, and entrepreneur in the fields of anticancer and anti-infective drug development. He published over 250 scientific papers over the course of his career and is listed as the inventor or coinventor on over 350 patents.

Certified as a personal fitness trainer by both the American Council on Exercise and the National Academy of Sports Medicine, Cook's continuing-education courses focus on physical fitness for older adults, including the frail and infirm.

www.ingramcontent.com/pod-product-compliance
Lightning Source LLC
Chambersburg PA
CBHW072211280526
45788CB00002B/978